MEDITERRANEAN DIET COOKBOOK FOR TYPE 2 DIABETES

The essential dietary guide with 50 quick and easy-to-prepare low-carb recipes for prevention and management of type 2 diabetics

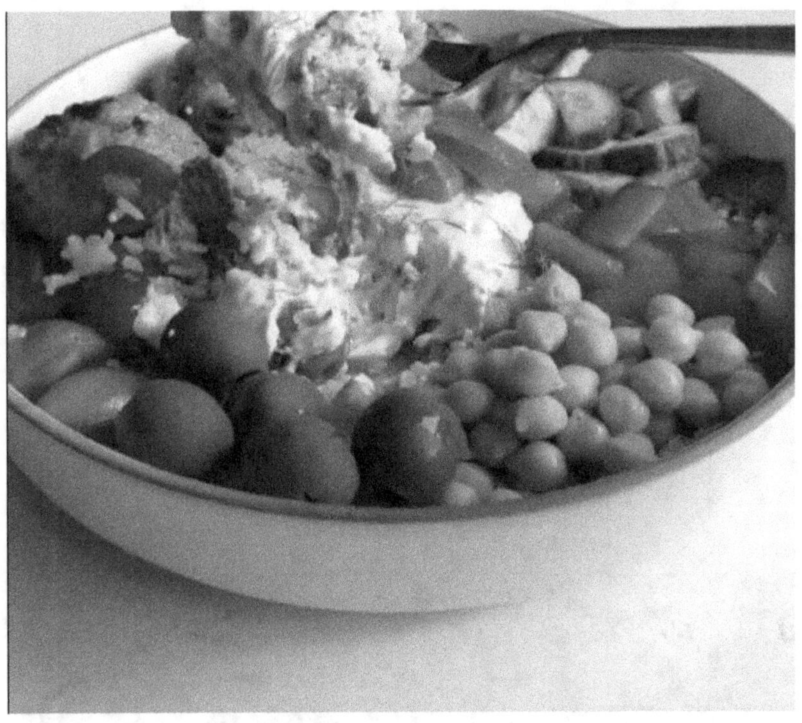

DR. COLE HULL

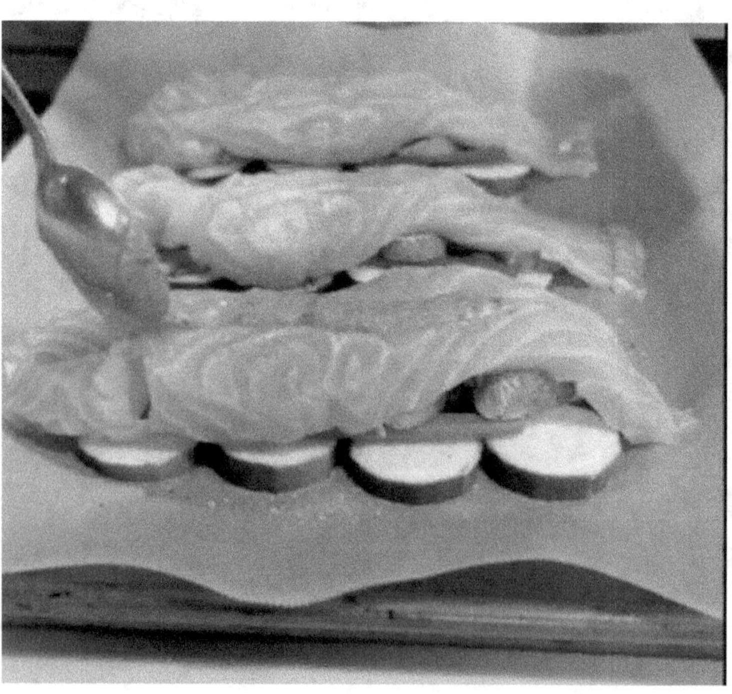

TABLE OF CONTENT

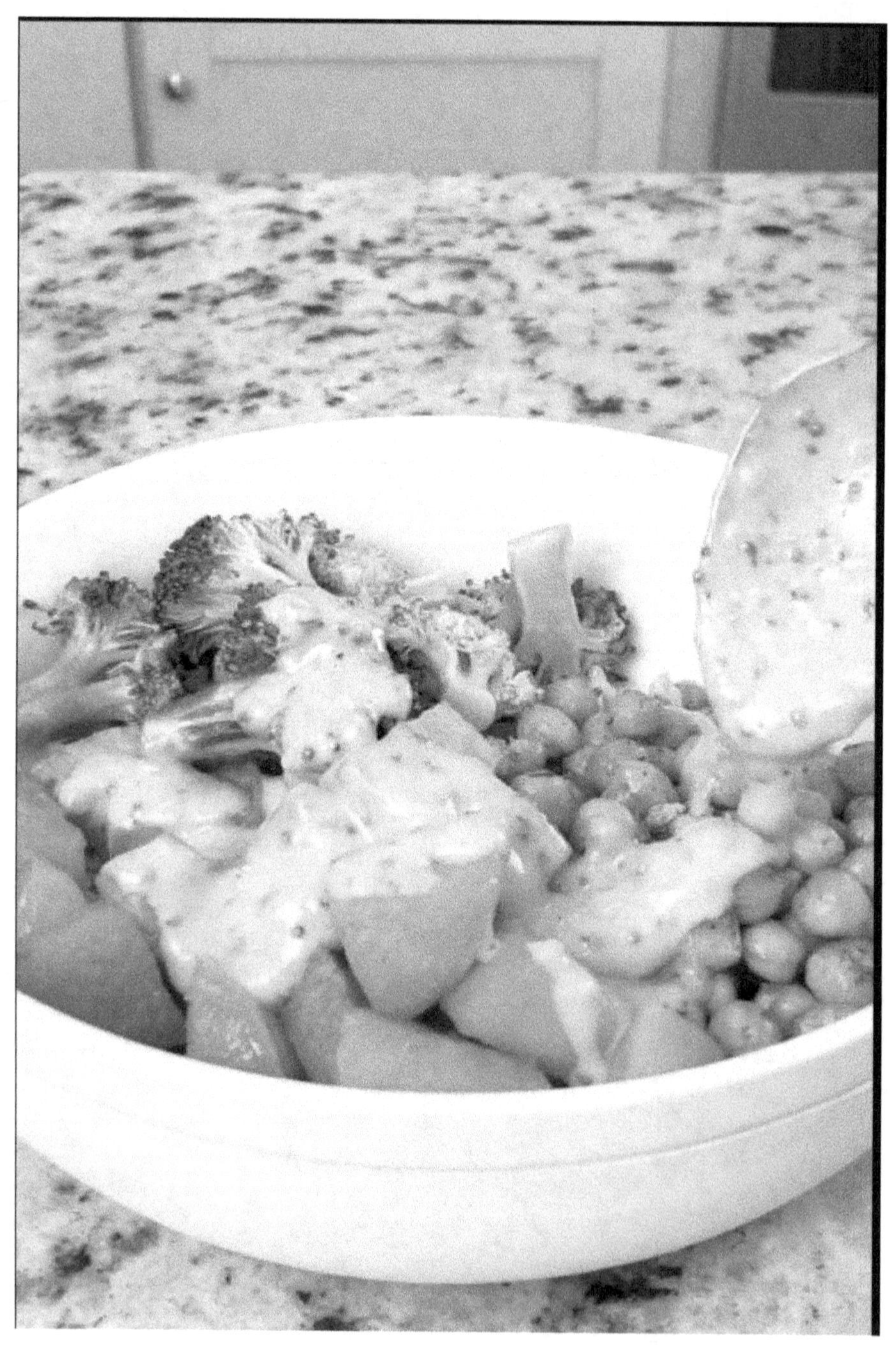

1. INTRODUCTION

The Mediterranean diet has been extensively studied for its benefits in managing type 2 diabetes and prediabetic states. Recent research, including systematic reviews and meta-analyses of randomized controlled trials (RCTs), emphasizes the effectiveness of the Mediterranean diet in both the prevention and management of type 2 diabetes.

Key findings from these studies highlight that the Mediterranean diet, known for its richness in fruits, vegetables, whole grains, and healthy fats, particularly olive oil, can positively impact blood sugar control. This diet has been shown to lead to improvements in glycosylated hemoglobin (HbA1c) levels, a key indicator of long-term blood sugar management in individuals with type 2 diabetes.

Additionally, the diet's potential for inducing remission from metabolic syndrome, which is a cluster of conditions including high blood pressure, high blood sugar, and abnormal cholesterol levels, has also been observed.

The mechanism behind the effectiveness of the Mediterranean diet in managing type 2 diabetes includes its anti-inflammatory and antioxidant properties, along with its influence on gut microbiota.

These factors collectively contribute to better glycemic control and overall metabolic health.

Moreover, the Mediterranean diet is not only beneficial for those already diagnosed with type 2 diabetes but also plays a significant role in preventing its onset. This is particularly important given the rising prevalence of type 2 diabetes globally, associated with lifestyle and dietary patterns.

In essence, the Mediterranean diet stands out as a beneficial dietary pattern for individuals with type 2 diabetes or at risk of developing it. Its comprehensive approach to improving various health markers, beyond just blood sugar levels, makes it a valuable tool in the management and prevention of type 2 diabetes and related metabolic conditions

Understanding Type 2 Diabetes

Type 2 diabetes is a chronic condition that significantly impacts the body's ability to regulate and use sugar (glucose) as fuel. This long-term condition results in elevated levels of sugar in the bloodstream, leading to various health complications if not managed effectively.

The underlying issues in type 2 diabetes involve resistance to insulin by cells in the muscle, fat, and liver, and the pancreas' inability to produce sufficient insulin to maintain healthy blood sugar levels. The exact reasons for these malfunctions are not entirely clear, but factors like being overweight, inactive, and genetic predispositions play pivotal roles.

Symptoms of type 2 diabetes can be mild and go unnoticed in some individuals. Common signs include increased urination, intense thirst, hunger despite eating, extreme fatigue, blurry vision, and slow-healing wounds. It's crucial for early detection and management to prevent the progression of the disease and its complications.

The risk factors for type 2 diabetes are multifaceted. Being overweight or obese significantly increases risk, as does the distribution of fat primarily in the abdomen. Physical inactivity, family history, certain racial and ethnic backgrounds, unhealthy cholesterol levels, older age, prediabetes conditions, gestational diabetes history, and polycystic ovary syndrome all contribute to the risk profile for developing type 2 diabetes.

Complications from unmanaged type 2 diabetes are serious and can affect many major organs, including the heart, blood vessels, nerves, kidneys, and eyes. It increases the risk of heart disease, stroke, neuropathy, kidney disease, and eye conditions. Additionally, it can slow wound healing and increase the risk of skin conditions and hearing problems.

Prevention and management of type 2 diabetes focus on lifestyle choices. A healthy diet low in fat and calories and high in fiber, regular physical activity, weight loss, and reducing periods of inactivity are key. For those with prediabetes, these changes can significantly lower the risk of progressing to type 2 diabetes. In some cases, medications like metformin are prescribed to help manage or prevent the condition.

Managing type 2 diabetes effectively involves regular check-ups with healthcare professionals, monitoring blood sugar levels, adopting a healthy lifestyle, and staying educated about the disease. It's also essential to be aware of how to manage day-to-day aspects of living with diabetes, like foot care, eye check-ups, and understanding the implications of high or low blood sugar levels.

The Role of Diet in Managing Type 2 Diabetes

Managing type 2 diabetes effectively requires a comprehensive approach, with diet playing a crucial role. This section explores the importance of diet in controlling this condition and the principles that guide dietary choices for diabetes management.

1. Principles of a Diabetes-Friendly Diet: Current guidelines emphasize the quality of macronutrients (types of carbohydrates, proteins, and fats), avoidance of processed foods, and adherence to healthy dietary patterns. Consistent evidence suggests the benefits of diets rich in vegetables, fruits, whole grains, legumes, and nuts, combined with regular physical activity.

It's important to understand that dietary advice for prevention and management should be aligned, with careful coordination with diabetes medications, especially in diets like very low-calorie or low carbohydrate ones.

2. Key Dietary Elements:
- *Whole Foods:* Focus on whole or unprocessed foods.

- ***Fiber:*** High-fiber foods help regulate blood sugar levels. Examples include vegetables, fruits, nuts, legumes, and whole grains.
- ***Heart-Healthy Fish:*** Consume fish like salmon and mackerel rich in omega-3 fatty acids, beneficial for heart health.
- ***Good Fats:*** Include monounsaturated and polyunsaturated fats found in avocados, nuts, and certain oils like olive and canola.
- ***Portion Control:*** Essential for managing energy intake.

3. Foods to Avoid: It's advised to reduce or avoid intake of processed red meats, refined grains, sugars (especially sugar-sweetened drinks), foods high in saturated and trans fats, cholesterol, and excessive sodium.

4. Weight Management: A core part of diabetes management is maintaining a healthy weight, as weight loss is linked to improvements in blood sugar levels, blood pressure, and lipid profiles.

5. Dietary Patterns: Diets like the Mediterranean diet are recommended for their beneficial effects in managing diabetes.

These diets emphasize foods high in nutritional value and low in processed and high-glycemic index ingredients.

6. Creating a Balanced Meal Plan: Utilize methods like the plate method, counting carbohydrates, and choosing foods based on the glycemic index to create a balanced diet plan. These methods help in maintaining a consistent blood sugar level.

7. Individualized Diet Plans: There is no one-size-fits-all diet for diabetes. The dietary approach should be tailored to individual needs, preferences, and cultural practices.

8. Research and Ongoing Developments: The field of dietary management in diabetes is continually evolving. Research into areas such as the impact of specific foods and macronutrient composition is ongoing to refine dietary recommendations further.

In short, diet is a cornerstone in managing type 2 diabetes. It involves understanding the right balance and types of foods, focusing on quality over quantity, and aligning dietary intake with overall diabetes management goals. A well-planned diet can help in controlling blood sugar levels, reducing the risk of complications, and improving overall health outcomes for individuals with type 2 diabetes.

Overview of the Mediterranean Diet

The Mediterranean Diet is based on the traditional eating habits of countries bordering the Mediterranean Sea. This diet is not a strict, standardized regimen, but rather a collection of eating styles influenced by cultural, religious, economic, and agricultural variations across different Mediterranean regions.

Health Benefits:

The Mediterranean Diet is recognized for its numerous health benefits, including the prevention of heart disease and stroke, reducing risk factors like obesity, diabetes, high cholesterol, and high blood pressure. This diet has been consistently ranked as one of the healthiest by various health organizations, including the American Heart Association. It's also known to improve brain health, potentially reducing the risk of dementia.

The diet emphasizes overall dietary quality, focusing on nutrient-dense foods and limiting those with high calories but little nutritional value. Unlike many trendy diets, the Mediterranean Diet is backed by scientific evidence for its long-term health benefits, particularly in cardiovascular health.

2. THE BASICS OF THE MEDITERRANEAN DIET

Key Components of the Mediterranean Diet

The Mediterranean Diet is a flexible and diverse eating plan based on the traditional foods of the countries surrounding the Mediterranean Sea. Its key components include:

1. Plant-Based Foods: The diet primarily revolves around vegetables, fruits, herbs, nuts, beans, and whole grains. These foods form the cornerstone of meals, providing essential nutrients and fiber.

2. Healthy Fats: A hallmark of the Mediterranean Diet is its focus on unsaturated fats, particularly olive oil, which is used as the main source of fat. Nuts and seeds also contribute healthy fats. These unsaturated fats help lower bad cholesterol levels and are beneficial for heart health.

3. Fish and Seafood: Regular consumption of fish, especially fatty fish like salmon, mackerel, and sardines, is encouraged due to their omega-3 fatty acid content. These fats are known for reducing inflammation and supporting heart health.

4. Moderate Protein Sources: The diet includes moderate amounts of dairy, poultry, and eggs. Red meat is consumed less frequently, emphasizing lean cuts when included.

5. Wine in Moderation: For those who consume alcohol, wine, especially red wine, is included in moderation. The diet acknowledges the cultural aspects of wine consumption but also recognizes the potential health risks associated with alcohol.

6. Minimally Processed Foods: Emphasis is placed on fresh and minimally processed foods, limiting the intake of processed and refined foods.

7. Portion Control and Balanced Meals: It advocates for mindful eating practices, portion control, and a balanced combination of food groups.

8. Physical Activity and Social Meals: The diet is not just about food; it also encompasses a lifestyle that includes regular physical activity and sharing meals with family and friends.

When starting the Mediterranean Diet, it's important to consider individual dietary needs and preferences. The diet can be adapted to be vegetarian or gluten-free, and while extra virgin olive oil is recommended for maximum benefits, regular olive oil can be a suitable alternative.

How the Mediterranean Diet Benefits Type 2 Diabetes

The Mediterranean Diet, with its focus on whole, minimally processed foods and healthy fats, offers significant benefits for individuals managing or at risk for type 2 diabetes (T2D). Here's how it helps:

1. **Improves Insulin Sensitivity:** The diet's emphasis on unsaturated fats, particularly from sources like olive oil and nuts, is associated with improved insulin sensitivity. The high concentration of polyphenols, antioxidant compounds present in Mediterranean diet foods, may also play a role in reducing insulin resistance, thus aiding in better blood sugar control.

2. Reduces Risk Factors: Adhering to the Mediterranean Diet can lead to a reduction in several risk factors associated with type 2 diabetes. The diet has proven benefits in mitigating cardiovascular risk factors which are often prevalent in individuals with diabetes. It also promotes an anti-inflammatory and antioxidative state in the body, contributing to overall metabolic health.

3. Supports Weight Management: Although not explicitly a weight-loss diet, the Mediterranean Diet's emphasis on nutrient-rich, fiber-dense foods can lead to satiety and reduced calorie intake, supporting weight management. Effective weight management is crucial in the prevention and management of type 2 diabetes.

4. Promotes a Holistic Lifestyle Change: Adopting the Mediterranean Diet goes beyond temporary dietary adjustments. It's about embracing a long-term, sustainable lifestyle change that includes healthy eating, physical activity, and mindful food choices. This holistic approach is beneficial for maintaining a healthy weight and managing blood sugar levels effectively.

5. Lowers the Risk of Other Diseases: In addition to being beneficial for managing diabetes, the Mediterranean Diet is linked to a lower risk of various other conditions, including certain types of cancers, Alzheimer's, and Parkinson's diseases.

6. Adaptable and Sustainable: The Mediterranean Diet is highly adaptable to individual preferences and needs. It can be modified to suit vegetarian or gluten-free requirements without losing its benefits. It's not a strict regimen but rather a flexible, enjoyable, and sustainable way of eating and living.

Switching to the Mediterranean Diet involves incorporating a variety of nutrient-dense foods into your meals, emphasizing whole grains, fresh fruits and vegetables, lean protein sources, healthy fats, and limiting the intake of processed and red meats, sweets, and high-fat dairy products.

It's essential to consult with healthcare professionals or dietitians when making significant changes to your diet, especially when managing a condition like type 2 diabetes, to ensure that the dietary plan meets your individual health needs and goals.

Foods to Embrace and Foods to Avoid in the Mediterranean Diet for Type 2 Diabetes

When adopting the Mediterranean Diet, especially for managing Type 2 Diabetes, it is crucial to understand which foods to embrace and which to limit or avoid.

Foods to Embrace:

1. *Whole Grains:* Include brown rice, quinoa, barley, bulgur, farro, buckwheat, and whole wheat products like bread and pasta.
2. *Nuts, Seeds, Beans, and Legumes:* Opt for almonds, walnuts, pistachios, cashews, sunflower seeds, sesame seeds, various beans, chickpeas, lentils, and peas.
3. *Vegetables and Fruits:* Emphasize a wide range of vegetables and fruits such as avocados, bell peppers, leafy greens, tomatoes, broccoli, cucumbers, as well as fruits like apples, berries, grapes, and citrus fruits.
4. *Healthy Fats:* Focus on healthy fats from sources like olives and olive oil.

5. ***Fish and Seafood:*** Incorporate fish like salmon, sardines, halibut, and mackerel, which are rich in omega-3 fatty acids.

6. ***Dairy, Eggs, and Poultry:*** Choose reduced-fat cheese, low-fat yogurt, and lean poultry like chicken and turkey.

7. ***Herbs and Spices:*** Use a variety of herbs and spices for flavoring instead of salt.

Foods to Limit:

1. ***Red and Processed Meats:*** Limit intake of beef, lamb, pork, and processed meats like sausages and hot dogs.

2. ***High-Fat Dairy Products:*** Cut back on whole and 2% milk, butter, margarine, and ice cream.

3. ***Sweets and Added Sugars:*** Reduce consumption of sweets, candies, and foods with added sugars.

Foods to Avoid:

1. ***Ultra-Processed Foods:*** Avoid chips, muffins, sugary cereals, and other heavily processed items.

2. ***Fast Food:*** Stay away from fast food options that are typically high in unhealthy fats and sugars.

3. ***Soda and Sweetened Drinks:*** Eliminate or greatly reduce the intake of sodas and other sugary beverages.

The Mediterranean Diet also encourages lifestyle elements like sharing meals with family, regular exercise, and, if alcohol is consumed, enjoying it in moderation. It's important to remember that this diet is about making a sustainable lifestyle change, not just a temporary adjustment to eating habits. For those managing Type 2 Diabetes, it's essential to monitor carb intake and control portions, especially for high-carb foods like pasta, potatoes, and rice.

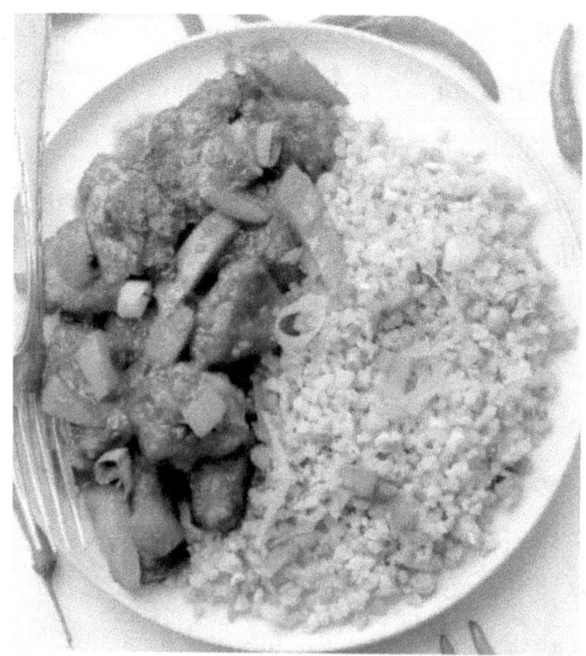

3. GETTING STARTED WITH THE MEDITERRANEAN DIET

Pantry Staples and Shopping Tips

When embarking on the Mediterranean diet, stocking your pantry with the right staples is crucial. Here are key items to include:

1. ***Grains:*** Opt for whole grains like brown rice, quinoa, couscous, bulgur wheat, and whole wheat pasta. These grains provide essential carbohydrates and fiber.

2. ***Canned and Jarred Items:*** Stock up on canned or jarred vegetables like artichokes, capers, olives, crushed tomatoes, and tomato sauce. These ingredients are versatile and convenient for quick meals.

3. ***Beans and Legumes:*** Include a variety of beans and legumes such as lentils, chickpeas, navy beans, and black-eyed peas. They're rich in protein and fiber.

4. ***Nuts and Seeds:*** Almonds, walnuts, pine nuts, and sesame seeds are great for snacking and adding texture to dishes.

5. ***Healthy Fats:*** Extra virgin olive oil is a staple. It's used in cooking and dressings for its health benefits and flavor.

6. ***Proteins:*** Canned fish like sardines and anchovies are economical and rich in omega-3 fatty acids. They're great for adding flavor to dishes.

7. ***Condiments:*** Keep red wine vinegar, balsamic vinegar, apple cider vinegar, and various herbs and spices. These enhance the flavor of your dishes without adding unhealthy elements.

8. ***Dairy:*** Choose reduced-fat or low-fat options like yogurt and cheese. These provide calcium and protein.

9. ***Fresh Produce:*** Emphasize fresh fruits and vegetables. They are the cornerstone of the Mediterranean diet.

When shopping, focus on fresh, unprocessed foods. The Mediterranean diet emphasizes the quality of ingredients, so choosing organic and locally sourced items where possible can enhance the nutritional value of your meals.

Kitchen Tools and Equipment Essentials

To successfully embrace the Mediterranean diet, having the right kitchen tools and equipment is essential. Here's a comprehensive list to get you started:

1. *Couscoussier:* This specialized pot is perfect for making homemade couscous, allowing you to steam it in the upper chamber while cooking a stew in the bottom pot.

2. *Measuring Cups:* Essential for accurately measuring both liquid and solid ingredients.

3. *Skewers:* Useful for Middle Eastern cuisine, particularly for cooking meats. Opt for stainless steel skewers for durability and repeated use.

4. *Tagine:* A traditional North African cooking pot, perfect for making slow-cooked, fragrant stews and dishes.

5. *Ibrik:* Essential for brewing authentic Turkish coffee.

6. *Mortar and Pestle:* Ideal for grinding spices and crushing garlic and herbs, enhancing the flavors in your dishes.

7. ***Wok:*** This versatile pan is excellent for stir-frying vegetables and meats, a common practice in Mediterranean cooking.

8. ***Wooden Cutting Board and Spoon:*** Necessary for chopping ingredients and stirring dishes without conducting heat.

9. ***Metal Bowls:*** Perfect for mixing ingredients, especially for dough preparations.

10. ***Colander:*** Useful for draining pasta, rice, or vegetables, and also for steaming.

11. ***Quality Knife Set:*** Including a chef's knife and various specialized knives for different purposes.

12. ***Non-Stick Skillet:*** Essential for cooking a variety of dishes without sticking.

13. ***Utensils like Spoons, Ladles, and Pallets:*** Choose materials that can withstand high temperatures and are gentle on non-stick surfaces.

Remember, having the right tools can make the process of preparing Mediterranean dishes more enjoyable and efficient. These tools not only aid in cooking but also help in bringing out the authentic flavors and textures that are characteristic of the Mediterranean diet.

Tips for Meal Planning and Preparation on the Mediterranean Diet

Meal Planning and Preparation Strategy

1. *Set Specific Goals:* Define what you want to achieve with your meal plan. For example, aim for a variety of breakfast options to avoid monotony, packable and satisfying vegetable-focused lunches, and quick, wholesome dinners.

2. *Nutritional Goals:* Balance is key. Ensure your plan includes a good mix of whole grains, vegetables, fruits, legumes, and healthy fats. Remember, the Mediterranean diet isn't restrictive but focuses on feel-good ingredients.

3. ***Batch Cooking:*** Prepare larger quantities of staples like whole grains or legumes ahead of time. This streamlines your cooking process throughout the week.

4. ***Versatile Ingredients:*** Choose ingredients that can be used in multiple dishes. For example, cooked chickpeas can be used in salads, bowls, or as a snack.

5. ***Meal Prep Steps:*** Allocate a couple of hours, typically over the weekend, to prep your meals. This could include tasks like roasting vegetables, cooking grains, and prepping proteins.

6. ***Storage:*** Store prepped ingredients in separate containers in the fridge. This makes it easy to assemble meals quickly.

7. ***Diverse Recipes:*** Incorporate a range of recipes to keep meals interesting. For instance, a mix of salads, grain bowls, and protein-rich dishes ensures a varied diet.

8. ***Use of Leftovers:*** Plan to use leftovers creatively. For instance, leftover roasted vegetables can be added to pasta dishes or salads.

9. *Flexible Approach:* Be adaptable with your meal plan. If something doesn't work one week, tweak it the next week. The goal is to find a rhythm that suits your lifestyle.

10. *Simplify Weeknight Cooking:* Even with meal prep, you might need to cook a bit during the week. Plan for quick and easy-to-assemble meals for busy nights.

Sample Meal Ideas

• *Breakfast:* Muesli with Greek yogurt and fresh fruit, savory breakfast toast with hummus and veggies.
• *Lunch:* Farro salad with arugula and walnuts, Greek salmon salad using leftover salmon.
• *Dinner:* Lemon garlic salmon with roasted broccoli, baked lemon chicken with toasted orzo and a Greek salad.

Remember, the Mediterranean diet is more about an overall eating pattern than strict rules, so feel free to adapt these tips and ideas to suit your personal preferences and lifestyle.

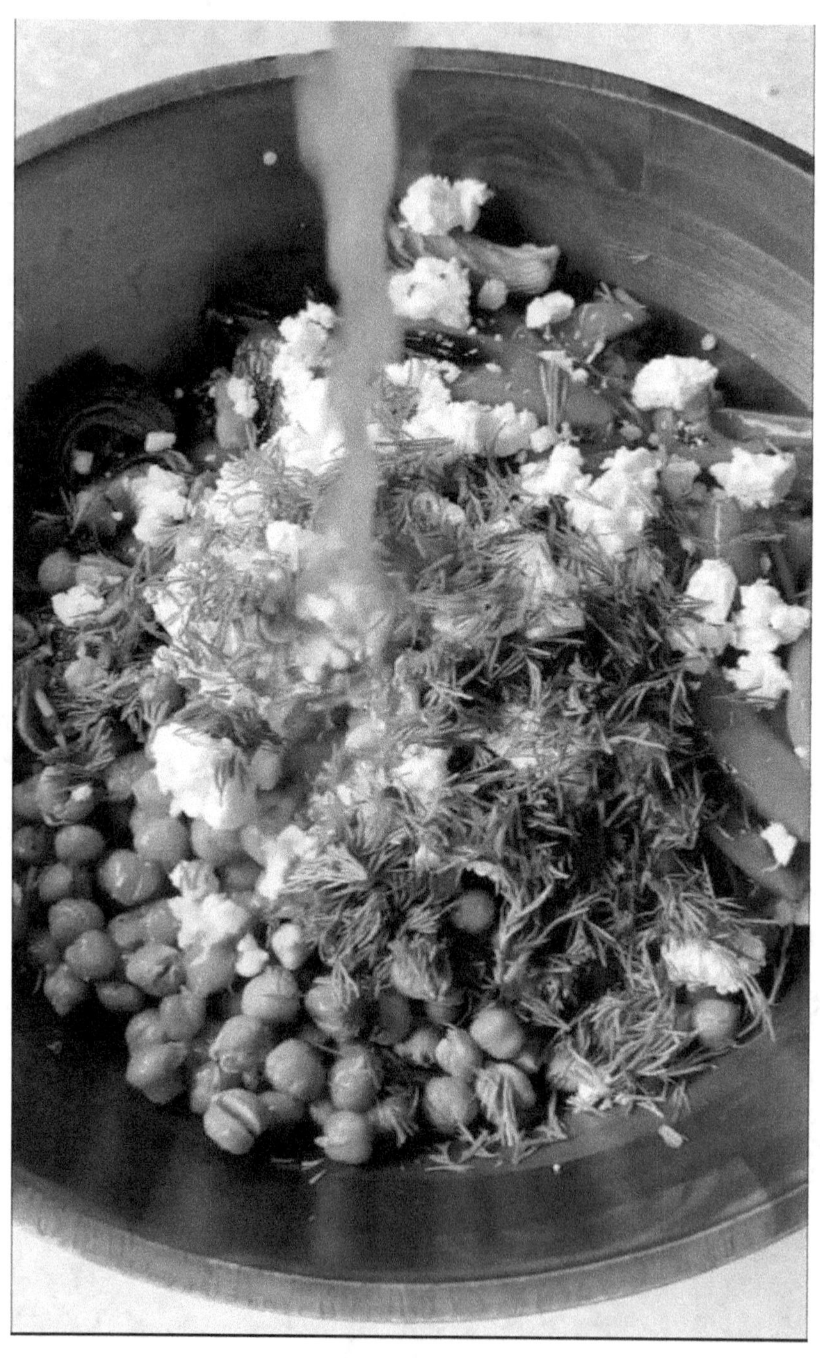

1. Spinach and Feta Omelette

Prep time: 5 minutes

Cook time: 10 minutes

Serving size: 1 omelette

Ingredients:

- 2 large eggs
- 1/4 cup fresh spinach, chopped
- 1/4 cup crumbled feta cheese
- 1/4 teaspoon dried oregano
- 1/4 teaspoon black pepper
- 1 teaspoon olive oil

Nutritional facts:

- Calories: 250 kcal
- Total fat: 20g
- Saturated fat: 8g
- Cholesterol: 385mg
- Sodium: 500mg

- Total carbohydrates: 3g
- Dietary fiber: 1g
- Sugars: 2g
- Protein: 16g

Preparation:

1. In a small bowl, whisk together the eggs, oregano, and black pepper.
2. Heat the olive oil in a non-stick skillet over medium heat.
3. Add the spinach to the skillet and cook for 1-2 minutes until wilted.
4. Pour the egg mixture into the skillet and cook for 2-3 minutes until the bottom is set.
5. Sprinkle the feta cheese over the top of the omelette and fold it in half.
6. Cook for an additional 1-2 minutes until the cheese is melted and the eggs are cooked through.

Health benefit:

This omelette is a great breakfast option for individuals with type 2 diabetes as it is low in carbohydrates and high in protein. The spinach provides a good source of fiber and vitamins, while the feta cheese adds a delicious flavor and a source of calcium. The use of olive oil instead of butter or margarine provides healthy fats that can help reduce the risk of heart disease, a common complication of diabetes.

2. Mediterranean Breakfast Quinoa

Prep time: 10 minutes
Cook time: 20 minutes
Serving size: 2 servings

Ingredients:

- 1/2 cup quinoa, rinsed
- 1 cup water
- 1/4 teaspoon salt
- 1/2 cup chopped fresh tomatoes
- 1/4 cup chopped cucumber
- 1/4 cup crumbled feta cheese
- 2 tablespoons chopped fresh parsley
- 1 tablespoon lemon juice
- 1 tablespoon olive oil
- 1/4 teaspoon ground black pepper

Nutritional facts (per serving):

- Calories: 280 kcal
- Total fat: 14g
- Saturated fat: 4g
- Cholesterol: 15mg
- Sodium: 360mg
- Total carbohydrates: 32g
- Dietary fiber: 4g
- Sugars: 3g
- Protein: 9g

Preparation:

1. In a saucepan, bring the quinoa, water, and salt to a boil. Reduce heat to low, cover, and simmer for 15 minutes or until quinoa is cooked.
2. In a bowl, combine cooked quinoa with tomatoes, cucumber, feta cheese, parsley, lemon juice, olive oil, and black pepper.
3. Toss well and serve either warm or chilled.

Health benefit:

This quinoa dish is ideal for type 2 diabetes patients as it provides a good balance of complex carbohydrates, protein, and healthy fats. The fiber in quinoa helps in blood sugar regulation, while the addition of fresh vegetables adds essential vitamins and minerals. Olive oil and feta contribute healthy fats that are beneficial for heart health.

3. Greek Yogurt Parfait with Nuts and Berries

Prep time: 5 minutes
Cook time: 0 minutes
Serving size: 1 serving

Ingredients:

- 1 cup Greek yogurt, unsweetened
- 1/2 cup mixed berries (strawberries, blueberries, raspberries)
- 1/4 cup mixed nuts (almonds, walnuts), chopped
- 1 tablespoon honey
- 1/4 teaspoon ground cinnamon

Nutritional facts:

- Calories: 320 kcal
- Total fat: 15g
- Saturated fat: 2g
- Cholesterol: 10mg

- Sodium: 60mg

- Total carbohydrates: 27g

- Dietary fiber: 4g

- Sugars: 18g

- Protein: 20g

Preparation:

1. In a serving bowl or glass, layer half of the Greek yogurt.

2. Add a layer of mixed berries, followed by a layer of chopped nuts.

3. Drizzle half of the honey and sprinkle a bit of cinnamon.

4. Repeat the layers with the remaining ingredients.

5. Serve immediately or chill in the refrigerator before serving.

Health benefit:

This parfait is a nutritious and satisfying option for type 2 diabetes patients. Greek yogurt provides a high-protein, low-carbohydrate base, while the berries offer antioxidants and fiber, which are important for managing blood sugar levels. Nuts add healthy fats and additional protein, making this a balanced meal to start the day.

4. Almond and Orange Oatmeal

Prep time: 5 minutes

Cook time: 10 minutes

Serving size: 1 serving

Ingredients:

- 1/2 cup rolled oats
- 1 cup almond milk
- 1/2 teaspoon orange zest
- 2 tablespoons sliced almonds
- 1 tablespoon honey
- 1/4 teaspoon ground cinnamon

Nutritional facts:

- Calories: 330 kcal
- Total fat: 12g
- Saturated fat: 1g
- Cholesterol: 0mg
- Sodium: 80mg
- Total carbohydrates: 48g
- Dietary fiber: 7g
- Sugars: 20g
- Protein: 10g

Preparation:

1. In a saucepan, bring the almond milk to a simmer.

2. Add the rolled oats and orange zest, and cook over medium heat for about 5 minutes or until the oats are tender.

3. Remove from heat and stir in the sliced almonds, honey, and cinnamon.

4. Serve warm, adding more almond milk if desired.

Health benefit:

This oatmeal recipe is particularly beneficial for those managing type 2 diabetes due to its high fiber content, which aids in blood sugar regulation. The inclusion of almonds provides healthy fats and additional fiber, while orange zest adds a refreshing flavor without excessive sugar. The overall combination makes for a balanced and heart-healthy breakfast option.

5. Avocado and Tomato on Wholegrain Toast

Prep time: 5 minutes

Cook time: 2 minutes

Serving size: 1 serving

Ingredients:

- 1 slice wholegrain bread
- 1/2 ripe avocado, mashed
- 1/2 tomato, sliced
- Salt and pepper, to taste
- 1/2 teaspoon lemon juice
- 1 tablespoon crumbled feta cheese (optional)

Nutritional facts:

- Calories: 250 kcal
- Total fat: 15g
- Saturated fat: 3g
- Cholesterol: 5mg
- Sodium: 300mg
- Total carbohydrates: 25g
- Dietary fiber: 7g
- Sugars: 5g
- Protein: 6g

Preparation:

1. Toast the wholegrain bread to your desired level.
2. In a small bowl, mix the mashed avocado with lemon juice, salt, and pepper.
3. Spread the avocado mixture over the toast.
4. Top with tomato slices and sprinkle with feta cheese, if using.
5. Serve immediately.

Health benefit:

This simple and quick breakfast option is excellent for type 2 diabetes patients. The wholegrain bread provides a source of complex carbohydrates and fiber, essential for blood sugar control. Avocado is a great source of healthy fats and fiber, while the tomato adds freshness and additional nutrients. This meal has a low glycemic index and is satisfying, helping to maintain steady blood sugar levels.

6. Baked Eggs in Avocado

Prep time: 5 minutes

Cook time: 15 minutes

Serving size: 2 servings

Ingredients:

- 1 ripe avocado, halved and pitted
- 2 eggs
- Salt and pepper, to taste
- 2 tablespoons shredded cheddar cheese
- 1 tablespoon chopped chives

Nutritional facts (per serving):

- Calories: 300 kcal
- Total fat: 25g
- Saturated fat: 6g
- Cholesterol: 185mg
- Sodium: 200mg
- Total carbohydrates: 8g
- Dietary fiber: 6g
- Sugars: 1g
- Protein: 12g

Preparation:

1. Preheat your oven to 425°F (220°C).
2. Scoop out a bit of avocado from each half to make room for the eggs.
3. Crack an egg into each avocado half. Season with salt and pepper.
4. Top each with shredded cheese and chives.
5. Bake in the preheated oven for about 15 minutes, or until the egg whites are set.
6. Serve warm.

Health benefit:

Baked eggs in avocado are a powerful breakfast for those with type 2 diabetes. The avocado provides healthy monounsaturated fats, which are beneficial for heart health. Eggs are a good source of protein, which helps in keeping you full and stabilizing blood sugar levels. This high-fiber, low-carb breakfast option is ideal for a diabetes-friendly diet.

7. Olive and Rosemary Focaccia

Prep time: 15 minutes (plus 1 hour for dough to rise)

Cook time: 20 minutes

Serving size: 8 pieces

Ingredients:

- 1 1/2 cups whole wheat flour
- 1 teaspoon instant yeast
- 1/2 teaspoon salt
- 1/2 cup warm water
- 2 tablespoons olive oil
- 1 tablespoon fresh rosemary, chopped
- 1/4 cup black olives, sliced
- Coarse sea salt, for sprinkling

Nutritional facts (per piece):

- Calories: 120 kcal
- Total fat: 5g
- Saturated fat: 1g
- Cholesterol: 0mg
- Sodium: 200mg
- Total carbohydrates: 16g
- Dietary fiber: 2g
- Sugars: 0g
- Protein: 3g

Preparation:

1. In a mixing bowl, combine flour, yeast, and salt.
2. Add warm water and 1 tablespoon olive oil, and knead into a soft dough.
3. Cover and let rise for 1 hour in a warm place.
4. Preheat oven to 400°F (200°C).
5. Press dough onto a baking sheet, forming a rectangle.
6. Dimple the dough with your fingers and drizzle with remaining olive oil.
7. Sprinkle with rosemary, olives, and coarse sea salt.
8. Bake for 20 minutes or until golden.
9. Cut into pieces and serve.

Health benefit:

Olive and Rosemary Focaccia is a hearty, fiber-rich option suitablefor type 2 diabetes patients. Whole wheat flour is a better option than refined flours due to its higher fiber content, which can help regulate blood sugar levels. The addition of olives and rosemary not only enhances flavor but also adds antioxidants. This recipe is lower in carbohydrates compared to traditional focaccia, making it more suitable for those managing diabetes.

8. Tomato and Cucumber Salad with Mint

Prep time: 10 minutes

Cook time: 0 minutes

Serving size: 2 servings

Ingredients:

- 1 large cucumber, diced

- 2 medium tomatoes, diced

- 1/4 cup red onion, finely chopped

- 2 tablespoons fresh mint, chopped

- 2 tablespoons olive oil

- 1 tablespoon lemon juice

- Salt and pepper, to taste

Nutritional facts (per serving):

Calories: 140 kcal

Total fat: 10g

Saturated fat: 1g

Cholesterol: 0mg

Sodium: 10mg

Total carbohydrates: 12g

Dietary fiber: 3g

Sugars: 6g

Protein: 2g

Preparation:

1. In a large bowl, combine cucumber, tomatoes, and red onion.
2. Add fresh mint, olive oil, and lemon juice. Toss to combine.
3. Season with salt and pepper according to taste.
4. Serve immediately or chill in the refrigerator before serving.

Health benefit:

This salad is a refreshing and hydrating choice for people with type 2 diabetes. The cucumbers and tomatoes are low in calories and carbohydrates, making them ideal for blood sugar management. The olive oil provides healthy fats, while the lemon juice and mint add flavor without additional sugar or sodium. This salad can aid in weight management, a key aspect of diabetes care.

9. Shakshuka with Spinach

Prep time: 10 minutes

Cook time: 20 minutes

Serving size: 2 servings

Ingredients:

- 1 tablespoon olive oil
- 1/2 onion, finely chopped
- 1 clove garlic, minced
- 1 bell pepper, chopped
- 2 cups fresh spinach
- 1 can (14 oz) diced tomatoes
- 1 teaspoon ground cumin
- 1 teaspoon paprika
- Salt and pepper, to taste
- 4 large eggs
- 2 tablespoons feta cheese, crumbled
- Fresh parsley for garnish

Nutritional facts (per serving):

- Calories: 300 kcal
- Total fat: 18g
- Saturated fat: 5g

- Cholesterol: 370mg

- Sodium: 600mg

- Total carbohydrates: 20g

- Dietary fiber: 5g

- Sugars: 10g

- Protein: 17g

Preparation:

1. Heat olive oil in a skillet over medium heat. Sauté onion and garlic until softened.
2. Add bell pepper and cook until tender.
3. Stir in spinach and cook until wilted.
4. Add diced tomatoes, cumin, paprika, salt, and pepper. Simmer for 10 minutes.
5. Create wells in the sauce and crack an egg into each well.
6. Cover and cook until eggs are done to your liking.
7. Sprinkle with feta cheese and parsley before serving.

Health benefit:

Shakshuka with spinach is an excellent breakfast for type 2 diabetes patients. It's rich in vegetables, providing ample fiber to regulate blood sugar levels. The protein from the eggs aids in satiety, reducing the likelihood of overeating. The spices, like cumin and paprika, not only add flavor but also contain anti-inflammatory properties beneficial for diabetes management.

10. Almond Porridge with Berries

Prep time: 5 minutes

Cook time: 10 minutes

Serving size: 1 serving

Ingredients:

- 1/2 cup rolled oats
- 1 cup almond milk
- 2 tablespoons almond butter
- 1/2 teaspoon vanilla extract
- 1 tablespoon honey
- 1/2 cup mixed berries (blueberries, raspberries)
- 1 tablespoon sliced almonds

Nutritional facts:

- Calories: 350 kcal
- Total fat: 15g
- Saturated fat: 1g
- Cholesterol: 0mg
- Sodium: 100mg

- Total carbohydrates: 45g
- Dietary fiber: 7g
- Sugars: 15g
- Protein: 10g

Preparation:

1. In a pot, combine rolled oats and almond milk. Bring to a simmer.
2. Cook for 5-7 minutes, stirring occasionally, until the oats are soft.
3. Stir in almond butter and vanilla extract.
4. Serve the porridge topped with honey, mixed berries, and sliced almonds.

Health benefit:

Almond porridge with berries is a diabetic-friendly breakfast that balances complex carbohydrates, protein, and healthy fats. The fiber in oats helps in regulating blood sugar levels. Almond butter provides healthy fats, which are important for heart health in diabetes management. Berries add natural sweetness and antioxidants without a significant increase in sugar content.

---

11. Lentil and Vegetable Soup

Prep time: 10 minutes

Cook time: 30 minutes

Serving size: 6 servings

Ingredients:

- Extra-virgin olive oil
- 1 medium yellow onion, finely chopped
- 4 large garlic cloves, minced
- 2 carrots, chopped
- 1 celery rib, chopped
- Kosher salt and black pepper
- 1 (28-ounce) can whole tomatoes
- 5 cups vegetable broth
- 1 dried bay leaf
- 1 tablespoon Italian seasoning
- ½ to 1 teaspoon red pepper flakes
- 1 cup green lentils, rinsed
- 2 cups baby spinach
- 1 cup chopped parsley leaves
- Splash red wine vinegar
- Freshly grated Parmesan cheese, for garnish (optional)

Nutritional facts (per serving):

- Calories: 161.8 kcal
- Carbohydrates: 30.5 g
- Protein: 10 g
- Fat: 0.7 g
- Saturated Fat: 0.1 g
- Fiber: 12.3 g
- Sugar: 5.9 g

Preparation:

1. Sauté onions, garlic, carrots, and celery in olive oil with salt and pepper until tender.
2. Add tomatoes, broth, bay leaf, seasoning, and lentils. Simmer until lentils are tender.
3. Stir in spinach, parsley, and vinegar. Serve with optional Parmesan cheese.

Health benefit:

This soup is a nutritious choice for type 2 diabetes due to its high fiber content from lentils and vegetables, which aids in blood sugar control. The lean protein from lentils supports satiety, while olive oil provides healthy fats beneficial for heart health.

12. Quinoa Greek Salad with Feta Cheese

Prep time: 15 minutes

Cook time: 15 minutes

Serving size: 4 servings

Ingredients:

- 1 cup quinoa
- 2 cups water
- 1 cucumber, chopped
- 1 cup cherry tomatoes, halved
- 1/2 red onion, thinly sliced
- 1/2 cup Kalamata olives, pitted and halved
- 1/2 cup feta cheese, crumbled
- 1/4 cup olive oil
- 2 tablespoons red wine vinegar
- 1 teaspoon dried oregano
- Salt and pepper to taste
- Fresh parsley, chopped, for garnish

Nutritional facts (approximate per serving):

- Calories: 350 kcal
- Carbohydrates: 40g

- Protein: 10g
- Fat: 18g
- Fiber: 5g
- Sugar: 3g

Preparation:

1. Cook quinoa in water as directed, then let it cool.
2. Combine cooled quinoa with cucumber, tomatoes, onion, olives, and feta cheese.
3. Mix olive oil, vinegar, oregano, salt, and pepper for the dressing.
4. Toss the salad with the dressing and garnish with parsley.

Health benefit:

This salad offers a balanced mix of complex carbohydrates, protein, and healthy fats, ideal for type 2 diabetes management. Quinoa is a low-glycemic grain that helps in blood sugar control. The fiber content from vegetables aids in digestion and satiety. The olive oil and feta cheese provide heart-healthy fats.

13. Grilled Chicken with Tzatziki Sauce

Prep time: 10 minutes (plus marinating time)
Cook time: 15 minutes
Serving size: 4 servings

Ingredients:

- 4 boneless, skinless chicken breasts
- 2 tablespoons olive oil
- 1 tablespoon lemon juice
- 1 teaspoon dried oregano
- Salt and pepper to taste
- For Tzatziki sauce:
- 1 cup Greek yogurt
- 1/2 cucumber, grated and drained
- 1 clove garlic, minced
- 1 tablespoon olive oil
- 1 tablespoon dill, chopped
- Salt and pepper to taste

Nutritional facts (approximate per serving):

- Calories: 300 kcal
- Carbohydrates: 4g

- Protein: 35g
- Fat: 15g
- Fiber: 1g
- Sugar: 3g

Preparation:

1. Marinate chicken in olive oil, lemon juice, oregano, salt, and pepper.
2. Grill chicken until fully cooked.
3. Mix Greek yogurt, cucumber, garlic, olive oil, dill, salt, and pepper to make tzatziki.
4. Serve chicken with tzatziki sauce on the side.

Health benefit:

Grilled chicken is a great source of lean protein, essential for blood sugar control in type 2 diabetes. The tzatziki sauce made with Greek yogurt adds probiotics and calcium, and the cucumber provides hydration and vitamins. This meal is low in carbohydrates and high in protein, making it suitable for diabetes management.

14. Chickpea and Roasted Pepper Salad

Prep time: 10 minutes

Cook time: 0 minutes

Serving size: 4 servings

Ingredients:

- 1 can chickpeas, drained and rinsed
- 1 cup roasted red peppers, sliced
- 1/2 red onion, thinly sliced
- 1/4 cup parsley, chopped
- 1/4 cup olive oil
- 2 tablespoons lemon juice
- 1 garlic clove, minced
- Salt and pepper to taste
- 1/4 cup feta cheese, crumbled

Nutritional facts (approximate per serving):

Calories: 250 kcal

Carbohydrates: 23g

Protein: 7g

Fat: 14g

Fiber: 6g

Sugar: 4g

Preparation:

1. Combine chickpeas, roasted peppers, red onion, and parsley in a bowl.
2. Whisk together olive oil, lemon juice, garlic, salt, and pepper for the dressing.
3. Toss the salad with the dressing and sprinkle with feta cheese.

Health benefit:

Chickpeas are a great source of fiber and protein, beneficial for regulating blood sugar and improving satiety. The addition of roasted peppers and onion adds antioxidants and vitamins. Olive oil provides healthy fats, and feta cheese adds calcium and flavor. This salad is a nutritious option for type 2 diabetes patients, offering a balance of nutrients without spiking blood sugar levels.

15. Mediterranean Tuna Salad

Prep time: 15 minutes

Cook time: 0 minutes

Serving size: 4 servings

Ingredients:

- 2 cans of tuna in olive oil, drained
- 1 cup cherry tomatoes, halved

- 1/2 cucumber, diced
- 1/4 red onion, thinly sliced
- 1/4 cup Kalamata olives, sliced
- 1/4 cup chopped fresh basil
- 2 tablespoons capers, drained
- 3 tablespoons olive oil
- 1 tablespoon lemon juice
- Salt and pepper to taste

Nutritional facts (approximate per serving):

- Calories: 200 kcal
- Carbohydrates: 5g
- Protein: 25g
- Fat: 10g
- Fiber: 2g
- Sugar: 2g

Preparation:

1. Combine tuna, tomatoes, cucumber, onion, olives, basil, and capers in a bowl.
2. Whisk together olive oil, lemon juice, salt, and pepper for the dressing.
3. Toss the salad with the dressing.

Health benefit:

Tuna provides a good source of omega-3 fatty acids, beneficial for heart health, which is crucial for type 2 diabetes patients. The salad's high protein and fiber content, coming from vegetables and tuna, help maintain stable blood sugar levels and provide satiety. This meal is low in carbohydrates and high in essential nutrients.

16. Stuffed Vine Leaves (Dolma)

Prep time: 30 minutes
Cook time: 60 minutes
Serving size: 6 servings

Ingredients:

- 1 jar grape leaves (about 30 leaves)
- 1 cup uncooked short-grain rice
- 1/2 cup olive oil
- 1 large onion, finely chopped
- 1/4 cup fresh dill, chopped
- 1/4 cup fresh parsley, chopped
- 1 tablespoon dried mint
- Juice of 2 lemons
- Salt and pepper to taste
- 2 cups vegetable broth

Nutritional facts (approximate per serving):

- Calories: 200 kcal
- Carbohydrates: 25g
- Protein: 4g
- Fat: 10g
- Fiber: 3g
- Sugar: 2g

Preparation:

1. Prepare the rice filling with olive oil, onion, dill, parsley, mint, and seasoning.
2. Wrap the filling in grape leaves.
3. Arrange in a pot and pour over vegetable broth and lemon juice.
4. Simmer for about an hour until the rice is cooked.

Health benefit:

Stuffed vine leaves are low in calories and high in fiber, making them suitable for diabetes management. The fiber from rice and grape leaves aids in blood sugar control, while the herbs provide antioxidants. This dish is heart-healthy due to the use of olive oil and offers a balanced mix of carbohydrates, protein, and fats.

17. Eggplant and Zucchini Caponata

Prep time: 15 minutes

Cook time: 30 minutes

Serving size: 4 servings

Ingredients:

- 1 large eggplant, diced
- 2 zucchinis, diced
- 1 red bell pepper, chopped
- 1 onion, chopped
- 2 cloves garlic, minced
- 1/4 cup olive oil
- 2 tablespoons red wine vinegar
- 1 can (14 oz) diced tomatoes
- 1/4 cup capers, drained
- Salt and pepper to taste
- Fresh basil for garnish

Nutritional facts (approximate per serving):

- Calories: 180 kcal
- Carbohydrates: 20g
- Protein: 3g
- Fat: 10g

- Fiber: 6g
- Sugar: 10g

Preparation:

1. Sauté eggplant, zucchini, bell pepper, onion, and garlic in olive oil.
2. Add vinegar, tomatoes, and capers. Simmer until vegetables are tender.
3. Season with salt and pepper, and garnish with basil.

Health benefit:

This caponata is a fiber-rich dish ideal for type 2 diabetes. The variety of vegetables provides essential nutrients and antioxidants. The fiber content helps in blood sugar regulation, and the olive oil adds healthy fats beneficial for cardiovascular health. This low-calorie dish is also great for weight management.

18. Falafel with Tahini Dressing

Prep time: 20 minutes (plus soaking time)
Cook time: 10 minutes
Serving size: 4 servings
Ingredients:

- 2 cups dried chickpeas, soaked overnight
- 1 onion, chopped

- 2 cloves garlic, minced
- 1/4 cup fresh parsley, chopped
- 1 teaspoon ground cumin
- 1 teaspoon ground coriander
- Salt and pepper to taste
- Oil for frying
- For Tahini Dressing:
- 1/4 cup tahini
- 2 tablespoons lemon juice
- 1 clove garlic, minced
- Water as needed
- Salt to taste

Nutritional facts (approximate per serving):

- Calories: 300 kcal
- Carbohydrates: 35g
- Protein: 10g
- Fat: 15g
- Fiber: 9g
- Sugar: 6g

Preparation:

1. Process soaked chickpeas, onion, garlic, parsley, and spices into a coarse mixture.
2. Form into balls and fry until golden.
3. Combine tahini, lemon juice, garlic, and water for the dressing.
4. Serve falafel with tahini dressing.

Health benefit:

Falafel is a great source of plant-based protein and fiber, beneficial for blood sugar control in type 2 diabetes. The chickpeas provide a low-glycemic carbohydrate option. Tahini, made from sesame seeds, offers healthy fats and additional protein. This dish is filling and nutrient-dense, supporting overall health and diabetes management.

19. Turkish Red Lentil Soup

Prep time: 10 minutes
Cook time: 30 minutes
Serving size: 4 servings

Ingredients:

- 1 cup red lentils, rinsed
- 1 onion, finely chopped

- 1 carrot, diced
- 1 tablespoon tomato paste
- 1 teaspoon paprika
- 4 cups vegetable broth
- 2 tablespoons olive oil
- Salt and pepper to taste
- Lemon wedges for serving

Nutritional facts (approximate per serving):

- Calories: 220 kcal
- Carbohydrates: 30g
- Protein: 12g
- Fat: 5g
- Fiber: 15g
- Sugar: 4g

Preparation:

1. Sauté onion and carrot in olive oil until softened.
2. Add tomato paste, paprika, lentils, and broth. Simmer until lentils are tender.
3. Blend soup until smooth, season with salt and pepper.
4. Serve hot with lemon wedges.

Health benefit:

Red lentil soup is an excellent choice for individuals with type 2 diabetes. Red lentils are a low-glycemic food, rich in fiber and protein, which helps in regulating blood sugar levels and provides sustained energy. The addition of vegetables enhances the nutrient content without adding excess carbohydrates.

20. Couscous Salad with Dried Apricots and Almonds

Prep time: 15 minutes

Cook time: 5 minutes

Serving size: 4 servings

Ingredients:

- 1 cup couscous
- 1 1/4 cups boiling water
- 1/2 cup dried apricots, chopped
- 1/2 cup almonds, sliced and toasted
- 1/4 cup fresh parsley, chopped
- 2 tablespoons olive oil
- 2 tablespoons lemon juice
- Salt and pepper to taste

Nutritional facts (approximate per serving):

- Calories: 280 kcal
- Carbohydrates: 40g
- Protein: 8g
- Fat: 10g
- Fiber: 4g
- Sugar: 10g

Preparation:

1. Pour boiling water over couscous, cover and let sit until water is absorbed.
2. Fluff couscous and add apricots, almonds, and parsley.
3. Whisk together olive oil, lemon juice, salt, and pepper for dressing.
4. Toss salad with dressing and serve.

Health benefit:

Couscous salad is a great lunch option for type 2 diabetes, providing a balanced mix of complex carbohydrates, protein, and healthy fats. Couscous is a whole grain that helps in blood sugar regulation, while apricots add natural sweetness and fiber. Almonds provide healthy fats and additional protein.

21. Grilled Salmon with Lemon and Dill

Prep time: 10 minutes
Cook time: 10 minutes
Serving size: 4 servings

Ingredients:

- 4 salmon fillets
- 2 tablespoons olive oil
- 1 lemon, juiced and zested
- 2 tablespoons fresh dill, chopped
- Salt and pepper to taste

Nutritional facts (approximate per serving):

- Calories: 250 kcal
- Carbohydrates: 1g
- Protein: 23g
- Fat: 16g
- Fiber: 0g
- Sugar: 0g

Preparation:

1. Marinate salmon in olive oil, lemon juice, zest, dill, salt, and pepper.
2. Grill on medium heat until cooked through.
3. Serve with additional lemon slices and dill.

Health benefit:

Grilled salmon is rich in omega-3 fatty acids, beneficial for heart health, which is crucial for type 2 diabetes management. The low carbohydrate content makes it ideal for blood sugar control. The addition of lemon and dill adds flavor without extra calories or carbs.

22. Chicken Tagine with Olives and Lemons

Prep time: 20 minutes
Cook time: 40 minutes
Serving size: 4 servings

Ingredients:

4 chicken thighs

1 onion, chopped

2 cloves garlic, minced

1 lemon, sliced

1/2 cup olives, pitted

1 teaspoon turmeric

1 teaspoon cumin

2 cups chicken broth

2 tablespoons olive oil

Salt and pepper to taste

Fresh cilantro for garnish

Nutritional facts (approximate per serving):

- Calories: 350 kcal
- Carbohydrates: 6g
- Protein: 25g
- Fat: 25g
- Fiber: 2g
- Sugar: 2g

Preparation:

1. Brown chicken in olive oil, remove from pan.
2. Sauté onion, garlic, and spices. Add chicken, broth, lemon, and olives.
3. Simmer until chicken is cooked through.
4. Garnish with cilantro before serving.

Health benefit:

This dish combines protein from chicken with healthy fats from olives, suitable for diabetes management. The spices provide anti-inflammatory benefits, and the lemon adds a refreshing flavor and vitamin C without increasing the sugar content significantly.

23. Vegetable Paella

Prep time: 15 minutes
Cook time: 30 minutes
Serving size: 4 servings
Ingredients:

- 1 cup Arborio rice
- 2 cups vegetable broth
- 1 onion, chopped
- 1 red bell pepper, chopped
- 1 cup frozen peas
- 1/2 cup artichoke hearts
- 2 cloves garlic, minced
- 1 teaspoon paprika
- 1/2 teaspoon saffron
- 2 tablespoons olive oil
- Salt and pepper to taste
- Lemon wedges for serving

Nutritional facts (approximate per serving):

- Calories: 280 kcal
- Carbohydrates: 45g
- Protein: 6g
- Fat: 8g
- Fiber: 4g
- Sugar: 3g

Preparation:

1. Sauté onion, bell pepper, and garlic in olive oil.
2. Add rice, broth, paprika, saffron, and simmer until rice is tender.
3. Stir in peas and artichokes, heat through.
4. Serve with lemon wedges.

Health benefit:

Vegetable paella is a fiber-rich meal that is low in fat and high in complex carbohydrates, making it an excellent choice for blood sugar management. The variety of vegetables provides essential nutrients and antioxidants, while the rice offers a steady source of energy.

24. Greek Moussaka

Prep time: 30 minutes

Cook time: 1 hour

Serving size: 6 servings

Ingredients:

- 2 large eggplants, sliced
- 1 lb ground lamb or beef
- 1 onion, chopped
- 2 cloves garlic, minced
- 1 can (14 oz) crushed tomatoes
- 1/4 cup red wine
- 1/2 teaspoon cinnamon
- 2 tablespoons olive oil
- For Béchamel sauce:
- 2 tablespoons butter
- 2 tablespoons flour
- 1 1/2 cups milk
- Nutmeg, a pinch
- Salt and pepper to taste

Nutritional facts (approximate per serving):

- Calories: 450 kcal
- Carbohydrates:25g
- Protein: 23g
- Fat: 28g
- Fiber: 5g
- Sugar: 8g

Preparation:

1. Fry eggplant slices, set aside.
2. Cook meat, onion, garlic, add tomatoes, wine, cinnamon, simmer.
3. Layer eggplant and meat sauce in a dish.
4. Make béchamel sauce, pour over layers.
5. Bake until golden.

Health benefit:

Moussaka offers a balance of protein, fiber, and nutrients. Eggplants are low in carbohydrates and high in fiber, suitable for blood sugar control. The meat provides protein, while the béchamel sauce adds calcium. It's a filling dish, providing balanced nutrition for diabetes management.

25. Baked Cod with Tomato and Olive Salsa

Prep time: 15 minutes

Cook time: 20 minutes

Serving size: 4 servings

Ingredients:

- 4 cod fillets

- 2 tomatoes, chopped

- 1/4 cup Kalamata olives, chopped

- 2 tablespoons capers

- 1 garlic clove, minced

- 2 tablespoons olive oil

- 1 lemon, juiced

- Salt and pepper to taste

- Fresh parsley, for garnish

Nutritional facts (approximate per serving):

- Calories: 200 kcal

- Carbohydrates: 5g

- Protein: 22g

- Fat: 10g

- Fiber: 2g

- Sugar: 2g

Preparation:

1. Preheat oven, place cod in a baking dish.
2. Mix tomatoes, olives, capers, garlic, olive oil, lemon juice.
3. Top cod with the salsa mixture.
4. Bake until cod is cooked through.
5. Garnish with parsley.

Health benefit:

Baked cod is a lean source of protein, excellent for managing blood sugar levels. The tomato and olive salsa provides healthy fats, vitamins, and antioxidants, enhancing heart health. This dish is low in carbohydrates and calories, making it an ideal dinner option for type 2 diabetes.

26. Seafood Risotto

Prep time: 20 minutes
Cook time: 30 minutes
Serving size: 4 servings

Ingredients:

- 1 cup Arborio rice
- 2 cups seafood stock
- 1 cup mixed seafood (shrimp, scallops, mussels)
- 1 onion, finely chopped

- 2 cloves garlic, minced

- 1/2 cup white wine

- 2 tablespoons olive oil

- Salt and pepper to taste

- Fresh parsley, for garnish

- Parmesan cheese, grated, for garnish

Nutritional facts (approximate per serving):

- Calories: 320 kcal

- Carbohydrates: 45g

- Protein: 15g

- Fat: 8g

- Fiber: 2g

- Sugar: 2g

Preparation:

1. Sauté onion and garlic in olive oil.

2. Add rice, cook until translucent. Deglaze with wine.

3. Gradually add seafood stock, stirring constantly.

4. Add seafood in the last 10 minutes of cooking.

5. Season with salt, pepper. Garnish with parsley and Parmesan.

Health benefit:

Seafood risotto is a good source of lean protein and omega-3 fatty acids, beneficial for heart health in diabetes management. The dish is balanced in carbohydrates and proteins, which aids in maintaining stable blood sugar levels.

27. Lamb Chops with Mint Pesto

Prep time: 15 minutes

Cook time: 10 minutes

Serving size: 4 servings

Ingredients:

- 8 lamb chops
- For Mint Pesto:
- 1 cup fresh mint leaves
- 1/2 cup olive oil
- 1/4 cup Parmesan cheese, grated
- 2 cloves garlic
- Salt and pepper to taste

Nutritional facts (approximate per serving):

- Calories: 400 kcal
- Carbohydrates: 2g

- Protein: 25g

- Fat: 32g

- Fiber: 1g

- Sugar: 0g

Preparation:

1. Grill lamb chops to desired doneness.

2. Blend mint, olive oil, Parmesan, garlic, salt, and pepper for pesto.

3. Serve lamb chops topped with mint pesto.

Health benefit:

Lamb is a rich source of high-quality protein and essential vitamins and minerals, important for muscle maintenance and overall health in diabetes management. The mint pesto adds fresh flavors without added sugars.

28. Ratatouille with Herbed Quinoa

Prep time: 20 minutes

Cook time: 40 minutes

Serving size: 4 servings

Ingredients:

- 1 eggplant, diced

- 2 zucchinis, diced

- 1 bell pepper, diced

- 1 onion, diced

- 2 tomatoes, diced

- 2 cloves garlic, minced

- 1 cup quinoa

- 2 cups vegetable broth

- 2 tablespoons olive oil

- Herbs (basil, thyme, oregano)

- Salt and pepper to taste

Nutritional facts (approximate per serving):

- Calories: 300 kcal

- Carbohydrates: 40g

- Protein: 8g

- Fat: 12g

- Fiber: 6g

- Sugar: 6g

Preparation:

- Sauté vegetables in olive oil with garlic and herbs.

- Cook quinoa in vegetable broth.

- Combine ratatouille with herbed quinoa.

- Season with salt and pepper.

Health benefit:

Ratatouille with quinoa is high in fiber and low in fat, making it an excellent choice for blood sugar control. The variety of vegetables provides essential vitamins and minerals, while quinoa adds protein and a complete amino acid profile.

29. Roasted Cauliflower with Tahini Sauce

Prep time: 10 minutes
Cook time: 25 minutes
Serving size: 4 servings

Ingredients:

- 1 large cauliflower, cut into florets
- 2 tablespoons olive oil
- Salt and pepper to taste
- For Tahini Sauce:
- 1/4 cup tahini
- 2 tablespoons lemon juice
- 1 clove garlic, minced
- Water to thin
- Salt to taste

Nutritional facts (approximate per serving):

- Calories: 180 kcal
- Carbohydrates: 15g
- Protein: 6g
- Fat: 12g
- Fiber: 5g
- Sugar: 4g

Preparation:

1. Toss cauliflower florets with olive oil, salt, and pepper. Roast until tender.
2. Mix tahini, lemon juice, garlic, water, and salt for sauce.
3. Serve cauliflower with tahini sauce drizzled over.

Health benefit:

Roasted cauliflower is a low-calorie, high-fiber food that's ideal for type 2 diabetes management. It's low in carbohydrates and high in nutrients. The tahini sauce adds healthy fats and flavor without adding excessive sugars.

30. Moroccan Spiced Chickpea Stew

Prep time: 15 minutes

Cook time: 30 minutes

Serving size: 4 servings

Ingredients:

- 2 cans chickpeas, drained and rinsed
- 1 onion, chopped
- 2 cloves garlic, minced
- 1 can (14 oz) diced tomatoes
- 2 carrots, chopped
- 1 teaspoon cumin
- 1 teaspoon paprika
- 1/2 teaspoon cinnamon
- 4 cups vegetable broth
- 2 tablespoons olive oil
- Salt and pepper to taste
- Fresh cilantro for garnish

Nutritional facts (approximate per serving):

- Calories: 250 kcal
- Carbohydrates: 35g
- Protein: 10g

- Fat: 8g

- Fiber: 10g

- Sugar: 6g

Preparation:

1. Sauté onion and garlic in olive oil.

2. Add spices, chickpeas, tomatoes, carrots, and broth.

3. Simmer until vegetables are tender.

4. Season with salt and pepper. Garnish with cilantro.

Health benefit:

This stew is rich in protein and fiber from chickpeas, making it a great option for blood sugar control in type 2 diabetes. The spices add flavor and anti-inflammatory benefits, while the vegetables provide essential nutrients and fiber.

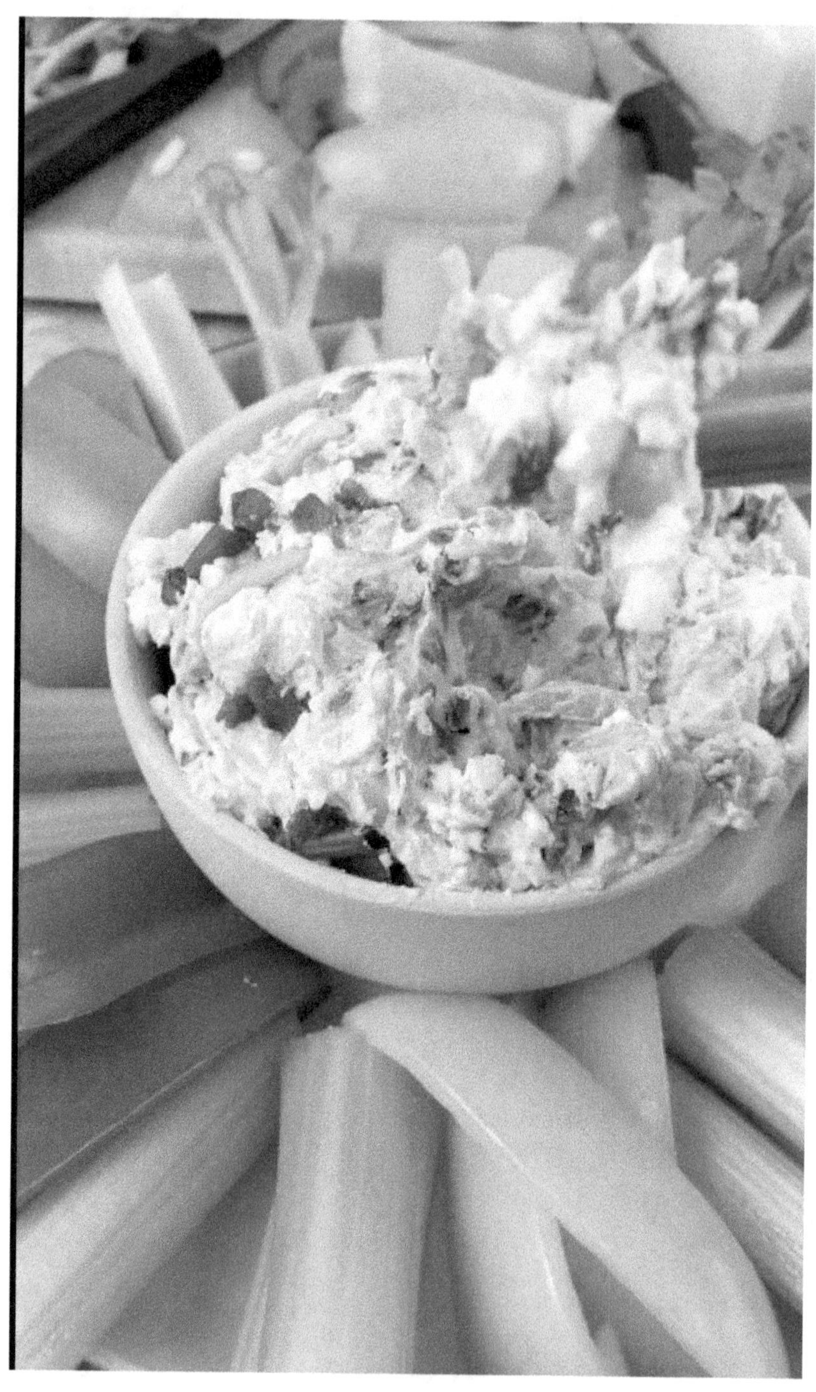

---

31. Hummus with Pita Bread

Prep time: 10 minutes

Cook time: 15 minutes

Serving size: 8 servings

Ingredients:

- 3 cups cooked chickpeas, peeled
- 1-2 garlic cloves, minced
- 3-4 ice cubes
- ⅓ cup tahini paste
- ½ tsp kosher salt
- Juice of 1 lemon
- Hot water (if needed)
- Extra virgin olive oil
- Sumac

Nutritional facts (approximate per serving):

- Calories: 150 kcal
- Carbohydrates: 20g
- Protein: 8g
- Fat: 5g

- Fiber: 6g
- Sugar: 3g

Preparation:

1. Puree chickpeas and garlic in a food processor.
2. Add ice cubes, tahini, salt, and lemon juice while blending.
3. Adjust consistency with hot water, blend until smooth.
4. Serve in a bowl with olive oil and sumac, accompanied by warm pita bread.

Health benefit:

Hummus, a protein and fiber-rich dish, is excellent for blood sugar control in type 2 diabetes. The fiber in chickpeas aids in digestion and satiety, while tahini provides healthy fats. It's a nutritious and filling snack or side dish.

32. Baba Ganoush

Prep time: 15 minutes
Cook time: 30 minutes
Serving size: 4 servings
Ingredients:

- 2 medium eggplants
- 3 tablespoons tahini
- 1 garlic clove, minced

- Juice of 1 lemon
- 2 tablespoons olive oil
- Salt and smoked paprika to taste
- Fresh parsley, chopped for garnish

Nutritional facts (approximate per serving):

- Calories: 180 kcal
- Carbohydrates: 15g
- Protein: 4g
- Fat: 12g
- Fiber: 7g
- Sugar: 6g

Preparation:

1. Roast eggplants until tender.
2. Scoop out the flesh and blend with tahini, garlic, lemon juice, and olive oil.
3. Season with salt and smoked paprika.
4. Garnish with parsley.

Health benefit:

Baba Ganoush is a low-carb, high-fiber dish beneficial for blood sugar control. The eggplant provides dietary fiber, while tahini adds healthy fats and protein, making it a nutritious choice for diabetes management.

33. Marinated Olives with Citrus Zests

Prep time: 10 minutes

Cook time: 0 minutes

Serving size: 6 servings

Ingredients:

- 2 cups mixed olives
- Zest of 1 orange
- Zest of 1 lemon
- 2 cloves garlic, minced
- 1/4 cup olive oil
- 1 teaspoon red pepper flakes
- Fresh thyme sprigs

Nutritional facts (approximate per serving):

- Calories: 150 kcal
- Carbohydrates: 3g
- Protein: 1g
- Fat: 15g
- Fiber: 2g
- Sugar: 0g

Preparation:

1. Combine olives, citrus zests, garlic, olive oil, red pepper, and thyme.
2. Marinate for several hours.
3. Serve as a snack or side.

Health benefit:

This snack is rich in healthy fats from olives and olive oil, beneficial for heart health in type 2 diabetes. The low carbohydrate content makes it a suitable snack for blood sugar control.

34. Feta and Watermelon Skewers

Prep time: 10 minutes
Cook time: 0 minutes
Serving size: 6 servings

Ingredients:

- 1/2 watermelon, cut into cubes
- 200g feta cheese, cut into cubes
- Fresh basil leaves
- Balsamic glaze for drizzling

Nutritional facts (approximate per serving):

- Calories: 120 kcal
- Carbohydrates: 15g
- Protein: 5g
- Fat: 5g
- Fiber: 1g
- Sugar: 12g

Preparation:

1. Thread watermelon, feta, and basil onto skewers.
2. Drizzle with balsamic glaze.
3. Serve chilled.

Health benefit:

The combination of watermelon and feta provides a balance of sweet and savory flavors, with a low-calorie count ideal for weight management in diabetes. Watermelon offers hydration and vitamins, while feta adds calcium and protein.

35. Roasted Red Peppers with Garlic

Prep time: 5 minutes

Cook time: 20 minutes

Serving size: 4 servings

Ingredients:

- 4 red bell peppers
- 4 cloves garlic, minced
- 2 tablespoons olive oil
- Salt and pepper to taste

Nutritional facts (approximate per serving):

- Calories: 110 kcal
- Carbohydrates: 12g
- Protein: 2g
- Fat: 7g
- Fiber: 3g
- Sugar: 6g

Preparation:

1. Roast peppers until charred, peel and slice.
2. Mix with garlic, olive oil, salt, and pepper.
3. Serve warm or cold.

Health benefit:

Roasted red peppers are low in carbohydrates and high in vitamin C, beneficial for overall health and immune support in diabetes management. The olive oil adds healthy fats.

36. Sun-dried Tomato and Basil Bruschetta

Prep time: 10 minutes
Cook time: 5 minutes
Serving size: 6 servings

Ingredients:

- 1 baguette, sliced
- 1/2 cup sun-dried tomatoes, chopped
- 1/4 cup fresh basil, chopped
- 2 cloves garlic, minced
- 1/4 cup olive oil
- Salt and pepper to taste
- Balsamic glaze for drizzling

Nutritional facts (approximate per serving):

- Calories: 180 kcal
- Carbohydrates: 20g

- Protein: 4g

- Fat: 9g

- Fiber: 2g

- Sugar: 3g

Preparation:

1. Toast baguette slices.

2. Mix tomatoes, basil, garlic, olive oil, salt, and pepper.

3. Top bread with mixture, drizzle with balsamic glaze.

Health benefit:

This bruschetta is a heart-healthy snack, rich in antioxidants from sun-dried tomatoes and basil. It's a low-calorie choice beneficial for blood sugar management.

37. Zucchini and Feta Fritters

Prep time: 15 minutes

Cook time: 10 minutes

Serving size: 4 servings

Ingredients:

2 zucchinis, grated

1/2 cup feta cheese, crumbled

1 egg

1/4 cup flour

2 tablespoons olive oil

1 clove garlic, minced

Salt and pepper to taste

Nutritional facts (approximate per serving):

- Calories: 150 kcal

- Carbohydrates: 10g

- Protein: 6g

- Fat: 9g

- Fiber: 1g

- Sugar: 3g

Preparation:

1. Mix zucchini, feta, egg, flour, garlic, salt, and pepper.
2. Form into patties, fry in olive oil.
3. Serve warm.

Health benefit:

These fritters are a good source of protein and fiber, ideal for diabetes management. Zucchini is low in calories, and feta adds calcium.

38. Garlic and Lemon Spinach

Prep time: 5 minutes

Cook time: 5 minutes

Serving size: 4 servings

Ingredients:

- 4 cups spinach
- 3 cloves garlic, minced
- 2 tablespoons olive oil
- Juice of 1 lemon
- Salt and pepper to taste

Nutritional facts (approximate per serving):

- Calories: 80 kcal
- Carbohydrates: 5g
- Protein: 3g
- Fat: 6g
- Fiber: 2g
- Sugar: 1g

Preparation:

Sauté garlic in olive oil.

Add spinach, cook until wilted.

Stir in lemon juice, season.

Health benefit:

Spinach is high in vitamins and minerals, especially beneficial for eye health in diabetes. The combination of garlic and lemon adds flavor without extra calories.

39. Stuffed Mushrooms with Herbs

Prep time: 15 minutes
Cook time: 20 minutes
Serving size: 4 servings

Ingredients:

- 12 large mushrooms, stems removed
- 1/4 cup breadcrumbs
- 1/4 cup Parmesan cheese, grated
- 2 tablespoons parsley, chopped
- 2 cloves garlic, minced
- 2 tablespoons olive oil
- Salt and pepper to taste

Nutritional facts (approximate per serving):

- Calories: 130 kcal
- Carbohydrates: 10g
- Protein: 6g

- Fat: 8g

- Fiber: 2g

- Sugar: 2g

Preparation:

- Mix breadcrumbs, cheese, parsley, garlic, salt, and pepper.

- Fill mushrooms with mixture, drizzle with oil.

- Bake until tender.

Health benefit:

Mushrooms are a low-calorie, nutrient-dense food, ideal for diabetes management. They're high in antioxidants and provide a good amount of protein when paired with cheese.

40. Artichoke and Olive Tapenade

Prep time: 10 minutes

Cook time: 0 minutes

Serving size: 6 servings

Ingredients:

- 1 can artichoke hearts, drained

- 1/2 cup olives, pitted

- 2 tablespoons capers

- 1 clove garlic

- 1/4 cup olive oil

- Juice of 1 lemon

- Salt and pepperto taste

- Zest of 1 lemon

- Fresh parsley for garnish

Nutritional facts (approximate per serving):

- Calories: 100 kcal

- Carbohydrates: 7g

- Protein: 2g

- Fat: 7g

- Fiber: 3g

- Sugar: 1g

Preparation:

1. Blend artichokes, olives, capers, garlic, olive oil, and lemon juice.

2. Season with salt, pepper, and lemon zest.

3. Serve garnished with parsley.

Health benefit:

This tapenade offers healthy fats from olives and olive oil, beneficial for cardiovascular health in diabetes. Artichokes are high in fiber and low in carbohydrates, making this a diabetes-friendly snack.

41. Greek Yogurt with Pistachios and Honey

Prep time: 5 minutes

Cook time: 0 minutes

Serving size: 1 serving

Ingredients:

- ¾ cup Greek yogurt
- 1-2 tsp honey
- 1 ½ tbsp chopped walnuts

Optional:

- ¼ medium apple, sliced
- ¼ tsp cinnamon

Nutritional facts (approximate per serving):

- Calories: 200 kcal
- Carbohydrates: 18g
- Protein: 10g
- Fat: 9g

- Fiber: 2g

- Sugar: 15g

Preparation:

1. Add yogurt to a bowl.

2. Top with walnuts or other nuts of your choice.

3. Drizzle with honey.

4. Optionally, add apple slices and sprinkle with cinnamon.

Health benefit:

This dish is a wholesome snack or dessert for type 2 diabetes. Greek yogurt is high in protein, aiding in blood sugar regulation. Nuts add healthy fats and fiber, while honey provides natural sweetness in moderation.

42. Baked Figs with Ricotta and Almonds

Prep time: 10 minutes

Cook time: 15 minutes

Serving size: 4 servings

Ingredients:

- 8 fresh figs, halved

- 1 cup ricotta cheese

- 1/4 cup almonds, chopped

- 2 tablespoons honey

- 1/2 teaspoon cinnamon

Nutritional facts (approximate per serving):

- Calories: 220 kcal

- Carbohydrates: 30g

- Protein: 10g

- Fat: 8g

- Fiber: 5g

- Sugar: 25g

Preparation:

1. Place fig halves on a baking sheet.
2. Top each with a spoonful of ricotta.
3. Sprinkle with almonds and cinnamon.
4. Drizzle with honey.
5. Bake until figs are warm and ricotta is slightly golden.

Health benefit:

Baked figs with ricotta offer a blend of natural sweetness, protein, and healthy fats. The figs provide fiber and essential nutrients, while ricotta adds protein and calcium, important for diabetes management.

43. Date and Walnut Balls

Prep time: 20 minutes

Cook time: 0 minutes

Serving size: 12 balls

Ingredients:

- 1 cup dates, pitted
- 1/2 cup walnuts
- 1/4 cup shredded coconut
- 1 teaspoon vanilla extract

Nutritional facts (approximate per serving):

- Calories: 100 kcal
- Carbohydrates: 15g
- Protein: 2g
- Fat: 4g
- Fiber: 2g
- Sugar: 12g

Preparation:

1. Blend dates and walnuts in a food processor until sticky.
2. Add vanilla extract and mix.
3. Form into balls and roll in shredded coconut.
4. Refrigerate before serving.

Health benefit:

These date and walnut balls are a healthy treat, providing natural sweetness, healthy fats, and protein. They are high in fiber, aiding in blood sugar control and digestive health.

44. Poached Pears in Red Wine

Prep time: 10 minutes

Cook time: 30 minutes

Serving size: 4 servings

Ingredients:

- 4 pears, peeled and cored
- 2 cups red wine
- 1/4 cup honey
- 1 cinnamon stick
- 1 orange, zest only

Nutritional facts (approximate per serving):

- Calories: 200 kcal
- Carbohydrates: 35g
- Protein: 1g
- Fat: 0g
- Fiber: 5g
- Sugar: 25g

Preparation:

1. Combine wine, honey, cinnamon, and orange zest in a saucepan.
2. Add pears and simmer until tender.
3. Serve pears with a bit of the poaching liquid.

Health benefit:

Poached pears are a light dessert option, perfect for diabetes management. The natural sweetness of the pears eliminates the need for added sugars, while the red wine adds antioxidants.

45. Chocolate-Dipped Strawberries

Prep time: 15 minutes

Cook time: 5 minutes

Serving size: 6 servings

Ingredients:

- 12 large strawberries
- 100g dark chocolate, melted
- 1/4 cup chopped nuts for garnish (optional)

Nutritional facts (approximate per serving):

- Calories: 120 kcal
- Carbohydrates: 15g

- Protein: 2g

- Fat: 7g

- Fiber: 3g

- Sugar: 10g

Preparation:

1. Dip strawberries in melted dark chocolate.

2. Optionally, roll in chopped nuts.

3. Refrigerate until chocolate sets.

Health benefit:

Chocolate-dipped strawberries provide a luxurious treat without a significant sugar spike. Dark chocolate is rich in antioxidants, and strawberries offer vitamins and fiber, making this a diabetes-friendly dessert.

46. Lemon and Olive Oil Cake

Prep time: 20 minutes

Cook time: 45 minutes

Serving size: 8 servings

Ingredients:

- 2 cups flour

- 3/4 cup sugar

- 1/2 cup olive oil

- 3 eggs

- Juice and zest of 1 lemon

- 1 teaspoon baking powder

- 1/2 teaspoon salt

Nutritional facts (approximate per serving):

- Calories: 300 kcal

- Carbohydrates: 40g

- Protein: 5g

- Fat: 15g

- Fiber: 1g

- Sugar: 20g

Preparation:

1. Mix flour, sugar, baking powder, and salt.
2. Whisk together olive oil, eggs, lemon juice, and zest.
3. Combine wet and dry ingredients. Pour into a greased pan.
4. Bake until a toothpick comes out clean.

Health benefit:

This cake uses olive oil as a healthier fat alternative, providing monounsaturated fats beneficial for heart health. The lemon adds a fresh flavor and vitamin C.

47. Orange and Almond Biscotti

Prep time: 15 minutes

Cook time: 40 minutes

Serving size: 15 biscotti

Ingredients:

- 2 cups flour
- 1 cup sugar
- 1/2 cup almonds, chopped
- 3 eggs
- Zest of 1 orange
- 1 teaspoon baking powder
- 1/4 teaspoon salt

Nutritional facts (approximate per serving):

- Calories: 140 kcal
- Carbohydrates: 20g
- Protein: 3g
- Fat: 5g
- Fiber: 1g
- Sugar: 10g

Preparation:

1. Combine flour, sugar, almonds, baking powder, and salt.
2. Mix in eggs and orange zest. Form a dough.
3. Bake as a loaf, then slice and bake again until crisp.

Health benefit:

These biscotti offer a good balance of carbohydrates and protein, with the almonds providing healthy fats. The orange zest adds flavor without extra sugar.

48. Pistachio Baklava

Prep time: 30 minutes
Cook time: 45 minutes
Serving size: 12 servings

Ingredients:

- 1 package phyllo dough
- 2 cups pistachios, chopped
- 1 cup butter, melted
- 1 cup honey
- Juice of 1/2 lemon
- 1 teaspoon cinnamon

Nutritional facts (approximate per serving):

- Calories: 350 kcal

- Carbohydrates: 40g

- Protein: 6g

- Fat: 20g

- Fiber: 3g

- Sugar: 25g

Preparation:

1. Layer phyllo dough with butter and pistachios.

2. Bake until golden. Pour over a mixture of honey, lemon juice, and cinnamon.

Health benefit:

While higher in sugar, this dessert can be enjoyed in moderation. Pistachios add protein and healthy fats, making it a more balanced option.

49. Ricotta and Honey Tart

Prep time: 20 minutes

Cook time: 30 minutes

Serving size: 8 servings

Ingredients:

- 1 pie crust
- 2 cups ricotta cheese
- 1/4 cup honey
- 3 eggs
- Zest of 1 lemon
- 1 teaspoon vanilla extract

Nutritional facts (approximate per serving):

- Calories: 280 kcal
- Carbohydrates: 30g
- Protein: 10g
- Fat: 14g
- Fiber: 0g
- Sugar: 15g

Preparation:

1. Blend ricotta, honey, eggs, lemon zest, and vanilla.

2. Pour into pie crust, bake until set.

Health benefit:

The tart features ricotta, a good source of protein and calcium, with honey adding natural sweetness. It's a calcium-rich dessert beneficial for bone health.

50. Apricot and Nut Bars

Prep time: 15 minutes
Cook time: 25 minutes
Serving size: 12 bars

Ingredients:

- 1 cup dried apricots, chopped
- 1 cup nuts (almonds, walnuts), chopped
- 1/2 cup whole wheat flour
- 1/4 cup honey
- 2 eggs
- 1/2 teaspoon cinnamon

Nutritional facts (approximate per serving):

- Calories: 150 kcal
- Carbohydrates: 15g
- Protein:5g
- Fat: 8g
- Fiber: 2g
- Sugar: 8g

Preparation:

1. Mix apricots, nuts, flour, honey, eggs, and cinnamon.
2. Press mixture into a baking pan.
3. Bake until set and golden.
4. Cut into bars.

Health benefit:

These bars offer a balance of natural sweetness from apricots and healthy fats from nuts. They're a fiber-rich snack, making them suitable for maintaining stable blood sugar levels in diabetes management.

9. 14-DAY MEDITERRANEAN DIET MEAL PLAN FOR TYPE 2 DIABETES

Day 1:

Breakfast: Spinach and Feta Omelette [Recipe 1]

Lunch: Quinoa Greek Salad with Feta Cheese [Recipe 12]

Snack: Hummus with Pita Bread [Recipe 31]

Dinner: Grilled Salmon with Lemon and Dill [Recipe 21]

Dessert: Greek Yogurt with Pistachios and Honey [Recipe 41]

Day 2:

Breakfast: Greek Yogurt Parfait with Nuts and Berries [Recipe 3]

Lunch: Lentil and Vegetable Soup [Recipe 11]

Snack: Baba Ganoush [Recipe 32]

Dinner: Chicken Tagine with Olives and Lemons [Recipe 22]

Dessert: Baked Figs with Ricotta and Almonds [Recipe 42]

Day 3:

Breakfast: Almond and Orange Oatmeal [Recipe 4]

Lunch: Mediterranean Tuna Salad [Recipe 15]

Snack: Marinated Olives with Citrus Zests [Recipe 33]

Dinner: Vegetable Paella [Recipe 23]

Dessert: Date and Walnut Balls [Recipe 43]

Day 4:

Breakfast: Shakshuka with Spinach [Recipe 9]

Lunch: Stuffed Vine Leaves (Dolma) [Recipe 16]

Snack: Feta and Watermelon Skewers [Recipe 34]

Dinner: Greek Moussaka [Recipe 24]

Dessert: Poached Pears in Red Wine [Recipe 44]

Day 5:

Breakfast: Avocado and Tomato on Wholegrain Toast [Recipe 5]

Lunch: Eggplant and Zucchini Caponata [Recipe 17]

Snack: Roasted Red Peppers with Garlic [Recipe 35]

Dinner: Baked Cod with Tomato and Olive Salsa [Recipe 25]

Dessert: Chocolate-Dipped Strawberries [Recipe 45]

Day 6:

Breakfast: Baked Eggs in Avocado [Recipe 6]

Lunch: Falafel with Tahini Dressing [Recipe 18]

Snack: Sun-dried Tomato and Basil Bruschetta [Recipe 36]

Dinner: Seafood Risotto [Recipe 26]

Dessert: Lemon and Olive Oil Cake [Recipe 46]

Day 7:

Breakfast: Olive and Rosemary Focaccia [Recipe 7]

Lunch: Turkish Red Lentil Soup [Recipe 19]

Snack: Zucchini and Feta Fritters [Recipe 37]

Dinner: Lamb Chops with Mint Pesto [Recipe 27]

Dessert: Orange and Almond Biscotti [Recipe 47]

Day 8:

Breakfast: Tomato and Cucumber Salad with Mint [Recipe 8]

Lunch: Couscous Salad with Dried Apricots and Almonds [Recipe 20]

Snack: Garlic and Lemon Spinach [Recipe 38]

Dinner: Ratatouille with Herbed Quinoa [Recipe 28]

Dessert: Pistachio Baklava [Recipe 48]

Day 9:

Breakfast: Almond Porridge with Berries [Recipe 10]

Lunch: Chickpea and Roasted Pepper Salad [Recipe 14]

Snack: Stuffed Mushrooms with Herbs [Recipe 39]

Dinner: Roasted Cauliflower with Tahini Sauce [Recipe 29]

Dessert: Ricotta and Honey Tart [Recipe 49]

Day 10:

Breakfast: Shakshuka with Spinach [Recipe 9]

Lunch: Lentil and Vegetable Soup [Recipe 11]

Snack: Zucchini and Feta Fritters [Recipe 37]

Dinner: Lamb Chops with Mint Pesto [Recipe 27]

Dessert: Apricot and Nut Bars [Recipe 50]

Day 11:

Breakfast: Avocado and Tomato on Wholegrain Toast [Recipe 5]

Lunch: Falafel with Tahini Dressing [Recipe 18]

Snack: Baba Ganoush [Recipe 32]

Dinner: Greek Moussaka [Recipe 24]

Dessert: Lemon and Olive Oil Cake [Recipe 46]

Day 12:

Breakfast: Baked Eggs in Avocado [Recipe 6]

Lunch: Mediterranean Tuna Salad [Recipe 15]

Snack: Hummus with Pita Bread [Recipe 31]

Dinner: Vegetable Paella [Recipe 23]

Dessert: Pistachio Baklava [Recipe 48]

Day 13:

Breakfast: Olive and Rosemary Focaccia [Recipe 7]

Lunch: Quinoa Greek Salad with Feta Cheese [Recipe 12]

Snack: Marinated Olives with Citrus Zests [Recipe 33]

Dinner: Baked Cod with Tomato and Olive Salsa [Recipe 25]

Dessert: Orange and Almond Biscotti [Recipe 47]

Day 14:

Breakfast: Greek Yogurt Parfait with Nuts and Berries [Recipe 3]

Lunch: Eggplant and Zucchini Caponata [Recipe 17]

Snack: Roasted Red Peppers with Garlic [Recipe 35]

Dinner: Chicken Tagine with Olives and Lemons [Recipe 22]

Dessert: Chocolate-Dipped Strawberries [Recipe 45]

This meal plan offers a variety of Mediterranean diet recipes, ensuring a balanced intake of nutrients. Each recipe is specifically selected to align with the dietary needs of type 2 diabetes patients, focusing on low glycemic index foods, high fiber, and healthy fats. Remember, portion control and regular physical activity are important aspects of diabetes management.

Tips for Adjusting the Meal Plan to Individual Needs

When using the 14-Day Mediterranean Diet Meal Plan, especially for managing type 2 diabetes, individualization is key. Here are some tips to tailor the plan to your specific needs:

1. *Assess Dietary Restrictions:* Consider any food allergies, intolerances, or specific dietary requirements you may have, and substitute or exclude ingredients accordingly.

2. *Monitor Portion Sizes:* Adjust portions to suit your caloric needs and blood sugar control goals. People with diabetes often need to pay special attention to carbohydrate portions to manage glucose levels effectively.

3. *Balance Your Plate:* Ensure each meal is balanced with a good mix of carbohydrates, proteins, and healthy fats. This balance is crucial for maintaining stable blood sugar levels.

4. *Stay Hydrated:* Drink plenty of water throughout the day. Hydration is important for overall health and can impact blood sugar levels.

5. ***Consider Meal Timing:*** Eating at regular intervals can help manage blood sugar levels. Plan your meals and snacks to fit into a consistent eating schedule.

6. ***Listen to Your Body:*** Pay attention to how different foods and meal timings affect your blood sugar levels. Continuous glucose monitoring or regular blood sugar testing can provide valuable feedback.

7. ***Exercise Impact:*** Consider the impact of physical activity on your blood sugar and adjust your meal plan as needed, particularly regarding carbohydrate intake around exercise times.

8. ***Consult Health Professionals:*** Regular check-ins with a dietitian or healthcare provider can help adjust the meal plan based on your health metrics, preferences, and lifestyle changes.

This personalized approach ensures the meal plan not only fits within the Mediterranean diet framework but also aligns with your unique health requirements and goals.

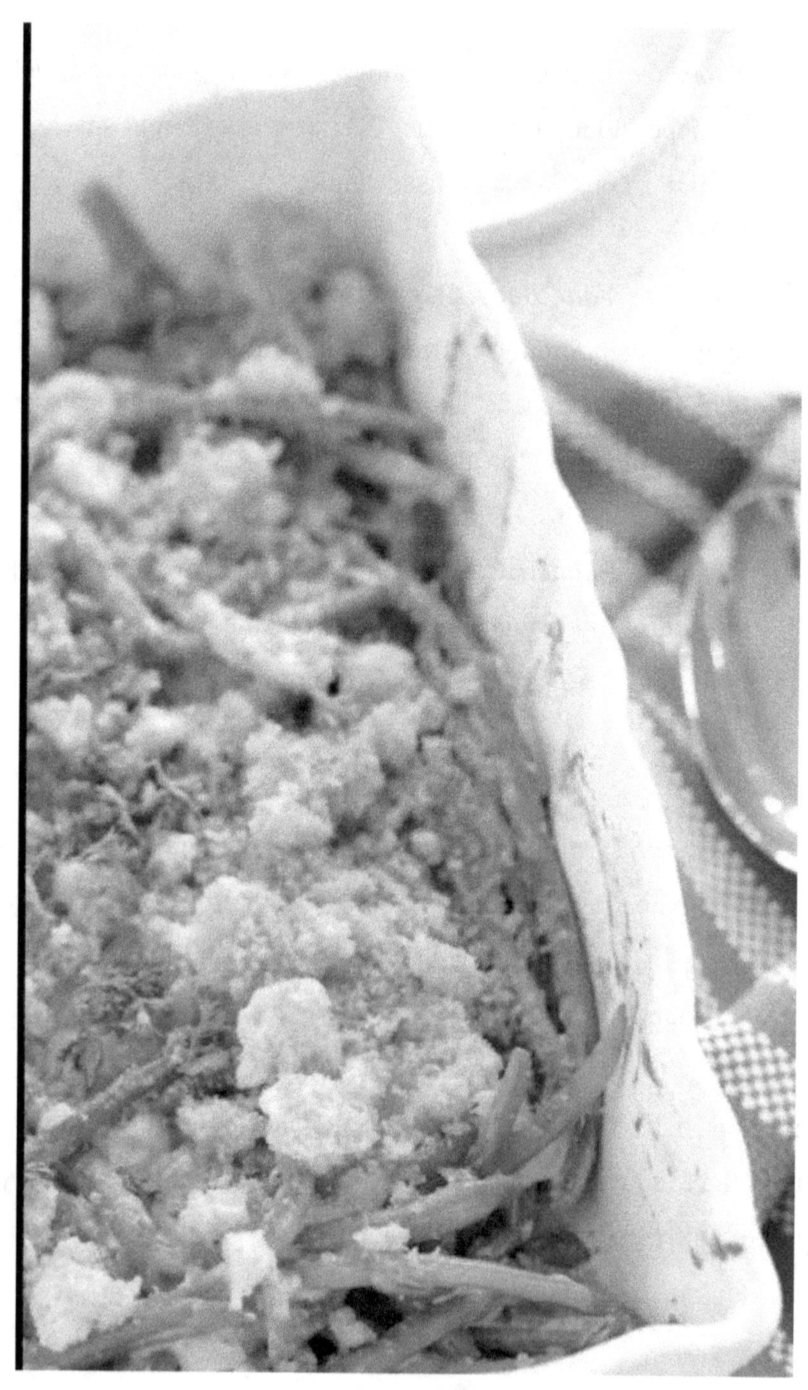

10. LIFESTYLE AND THE MEDITERRANEAN DIET

Incorporating Physical Activity

In the context of the "Mediterranean Diet for Type 2 Diabetes," integrating physical activity into daily life is essential. Exercise plays a pivotal role in managing diabetes and enhancing the effectiveness of the diet.

1. Regular Exercise: Aim for at least 150 minutes of moderate aerobic activity per week. This could include brisk walking, swimming, or cycling. Regular exercise helps improve blood sugar control, boosts cardiovascular health, and aids in weight management.

2. Strength Training: Incorporating strength training exercises at least twice a week can enhance muscle strength and improve insulin sensitivity. This could be through bodyweight exercises, resistance bands, or weights.

3. Flexibility and Balance: Practices like yoga or Tai Chi can improve flexibility, balance, and mental well-being, contributing to overall diabetes management.

4. Daily Movement: Incorporate more movement into your day-to-day activities. Take the stairs instead of the elevator, walk or cycle for short trips, and stand up or take short walks if you have a sedentary job.

5. Monitor Blood Sugar Levels: Pay attention to how your body responds to exercise. Some activities may require adjustments in food intake or medication to maintain stable blood sugar levels.

6. Enjoyment is Key: Choose activities you enjoy to ensure consistency and long-term adherence. Enjoyable exercise is more likely to become a regular part of your lifestyle.

Physical activity, as part of the Mediterranean lifestyle, enhances overall health and is especially beneficial for those managing type 2 diabetes. It complements the diet by helping to regulate blood sugar levels, reduce stress, and improve physical and mental health.

Stress Management and Mindful Eating

The Mediterranean Diet, when integrated into a lifestyle for managing Type 2 Diabetes, also emphasizes the importance of stress management and mindful eating.

1. Understanding Stress Impact: Chronic stress can negatively impact blood sugar levels and overall health. It's crucial to recognize stressors and address them proactively.

2. Relaxation Techniques: Incorporate relaxation practices like deep breathing, meditation, or yoga. These methods can reduce stress hormones which influence glucose levels.

3. Mindful Eating: Pay attention to what and how you eat. Eating mindfully involves savoring each bite, eating slowly, and listening to your body's hunger and fullness cues. This approach can prevent overeating and help in making healthier food choices.

4. Balanced Lifestyle: Balance work, leisure, and family life. Engaging in hobbies, spending time with loved ones, and ensuring adequate rest are integral to a holistic approach to health.

5. Connection Between Mind and Body: Recognize the relationship between emotional well-being and physical health. Emotional disturbances can affect dietary choices and vice versa.

6. Seek Support: Don't hesitate to seek professional help if stress becomes overwhelming. Counseling or support groups for diabetes management can be very beneficial.

Incorporating these practices along with the Mediterranean diet can lead to better management of type 2 diabetes, by not only focusing on what you eat but also how you eat and manage your overall well-being.

The Role of Community and Social Eating

In the Mediterranean Diet for Type 2 Diabetes, community and social eating play a vital role.

1. Shared Meals: Eating with family or friends not only enhances the enjoyment of food but also encourages healthier eating habits. Shared meals often lead to more balanced, diverse, and moderate food choices.

2. Cultural Connection: The Mediterranean diet is deeply rooted in cultural traditions which include social interactions around meals. This aspect helps in creating a positive relationship with food and eating.

3. Support System: Having a support system can aid in maintaining dietary changes and managing diabetes. Family and friends can provide encouragement and accountability.

4. Learning Opportunity: Social settings are great for exchanging recipes, cooking methods, and tips about the Mediterranean lifestyle. This communal learning can enrich your dietary approach.

5. Mindfulness and Appreciation: Eating with others often slows down the pace of meals, encouraging more mindful eating. It also enhances the appreciation of food's flavors, textures, and aromas.

Incorporating the social aspect of eating into the Mediterranean diet approach provides emotional support, enriches the eating experience, and contributes to the overall effectiveness of the diet in managing type 2 diabetes.

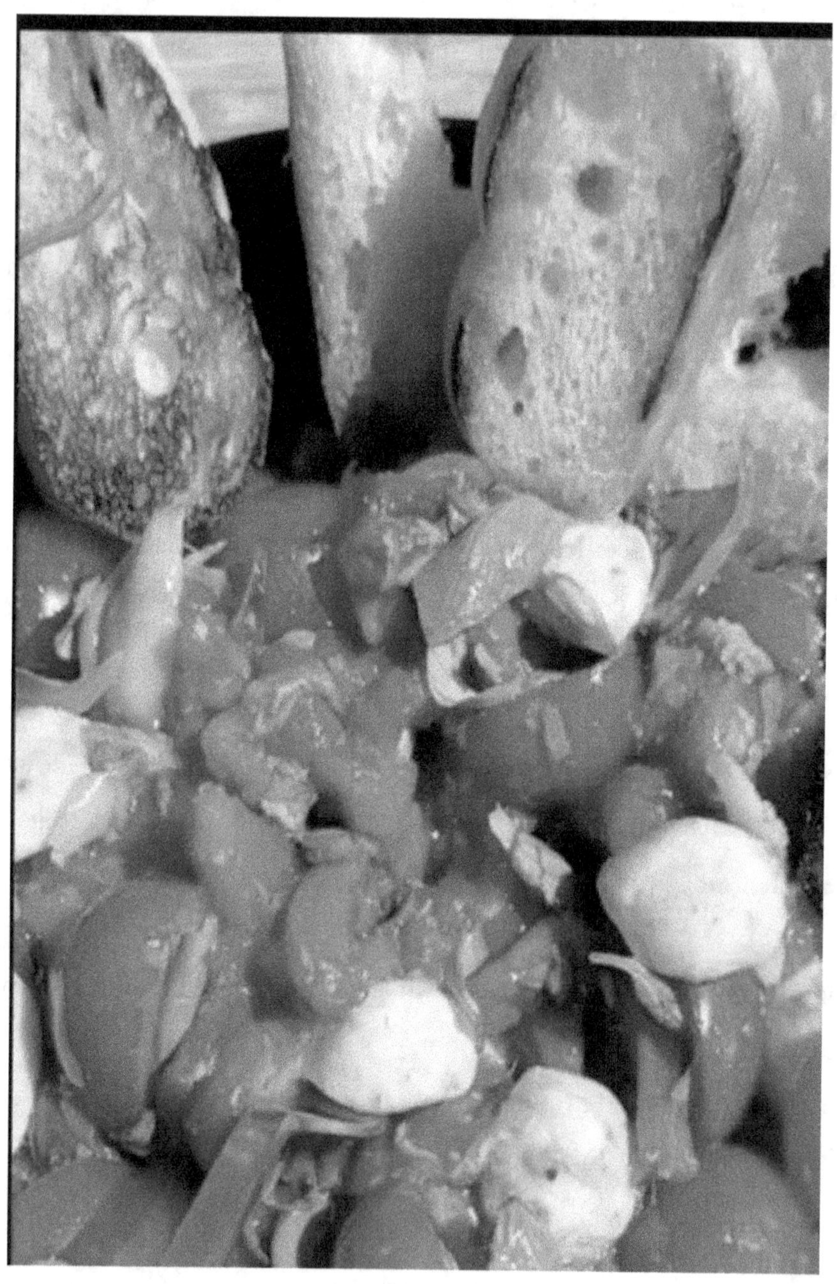

11. NAVIGATING CHALLENGES AND STAYING MOTIVATED

Eating Out and Social Events

Adhering to the Mediterranean Diet for Type 2 Diabetes while eating out or attending social events can be challenging. Here are some strategies:

1. **Menu Research:** Before dining out, review the restaurant's menu online. Look for dishes that align with the Mediterranean diet principles, such as grilled fish, salads, and vegetable-centric meals.

2. **Communicate Dietary Preferences:** Don't hesitate to ask for modifications to dishes, like dressing on the side or substituting fried items with grilled options.

3. **Portion Control:** Be mindful of portion sizes. You can share a dish or ask for a half portion if the servings are large.

4. **Healthy Choices at Social Events:** At social gatherings, focus on the healthier options available. Fresh fruits, vegetables, nuts,

and whole grains are often part of the spread and fit well with the diet.

5. Avoiding Temptation: It's easy to be tempted by unhealthy choices. Stay focused on your health goals, and remember how the foods you eat affect your diabetes management.

6. Drinking in Moderation: If you consume alcohol, do so in moderation. Opt for a glass of red wine, which aligns with the Mediterranean diet.

By planning ahead and making informed choices, you can enjoy eating out and attending social events without compromising your dietary goals.

Adjusting Recipes for Family and Friends

When following the Mediterranean Diet for Type 2 Diabetes, preparing meals for family and friends can present unique challenges. Here are some strategies:

1. Incorporate Familiar Elements: Modify recipes to include familiar ingredients that your family and friends enjoy while adhering to the Mediterranean diet principles.

2. Educate and Involve: Educate your loved ones about the benefits of the Mediterranean diet, especially in relation to diabetes management. Involve them in meal planning and preparation to make it a shared experience.

3. Balance and Variety: Offer a variety of dishes that cater to different tastes but still fit within the diet. This could include a mix of meat-based, vegetarian, and seafood options.

4. Healthy Substitutions: Make simple substitutions in traditional recipes, like using whole grains instead of refined grains, or olive oil instead of butter.

5. Focus on Flavor: Highlight the natural flavors of food with herbs, spices, and healthy fats like olive oil. This approach can make the dishes appealing to everyone, regardless of their diet.

By making these adjustments, you can enjoy meals with your family and friends without compromising your dietary needs.

Long-term Adherence to the Mediterranean Diet

Maintaining long-term adherence to the Mediterranean Diet, especially for managing Type 2 Diabetes, requires sustainable lifestyle changes:

1. Gradual Changes: Start with small, manageable changes to your diet and gradually incorporate more elements of the Mediterranean diet.

2. Enjoy the Journey: Focus on the variety, flavors, and enjoyment of Mediterranean foods. This diet is about pleasure in healthy eating, not restriction.

3. Set Realistic Goals: Set achievable goals and track your progress. Celebrate milestones to stay motivated.

4. Seek Support: Connect with others who are also following the Mediterranean diet. Support groups or online communities can provide encouragement and tips.

5. Be Flexible: The Mediterranean diet is adaptable. If you slip up, don't be too hard on yourself. The key is consistency, not perfection.

6. Educate Yourself Continuously: Stay informed about the diet and its benefits for diabetes management. This knowledge can reinforce your commitment and help you make informed choices.

By embracing these strategies, you can successfully adhere to the Mediterranean Diet over the long term, enjoying its health benefits and its role in managing Type 2 Diabetes.

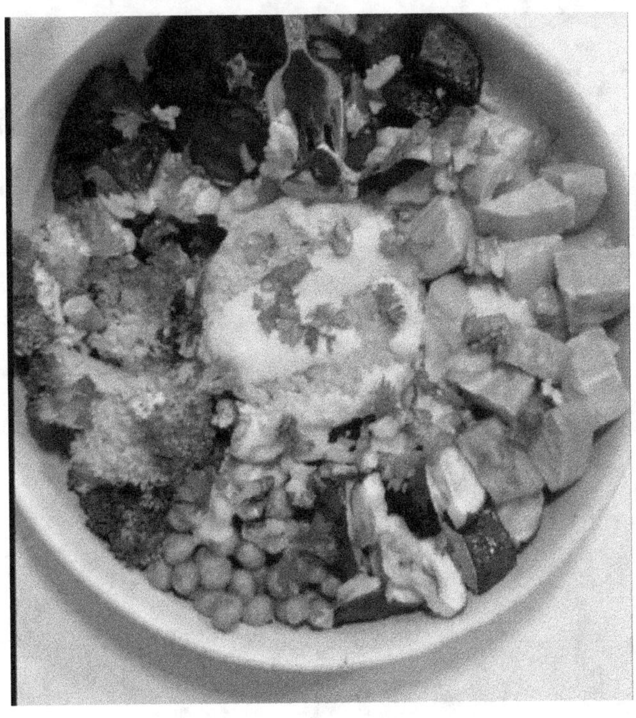

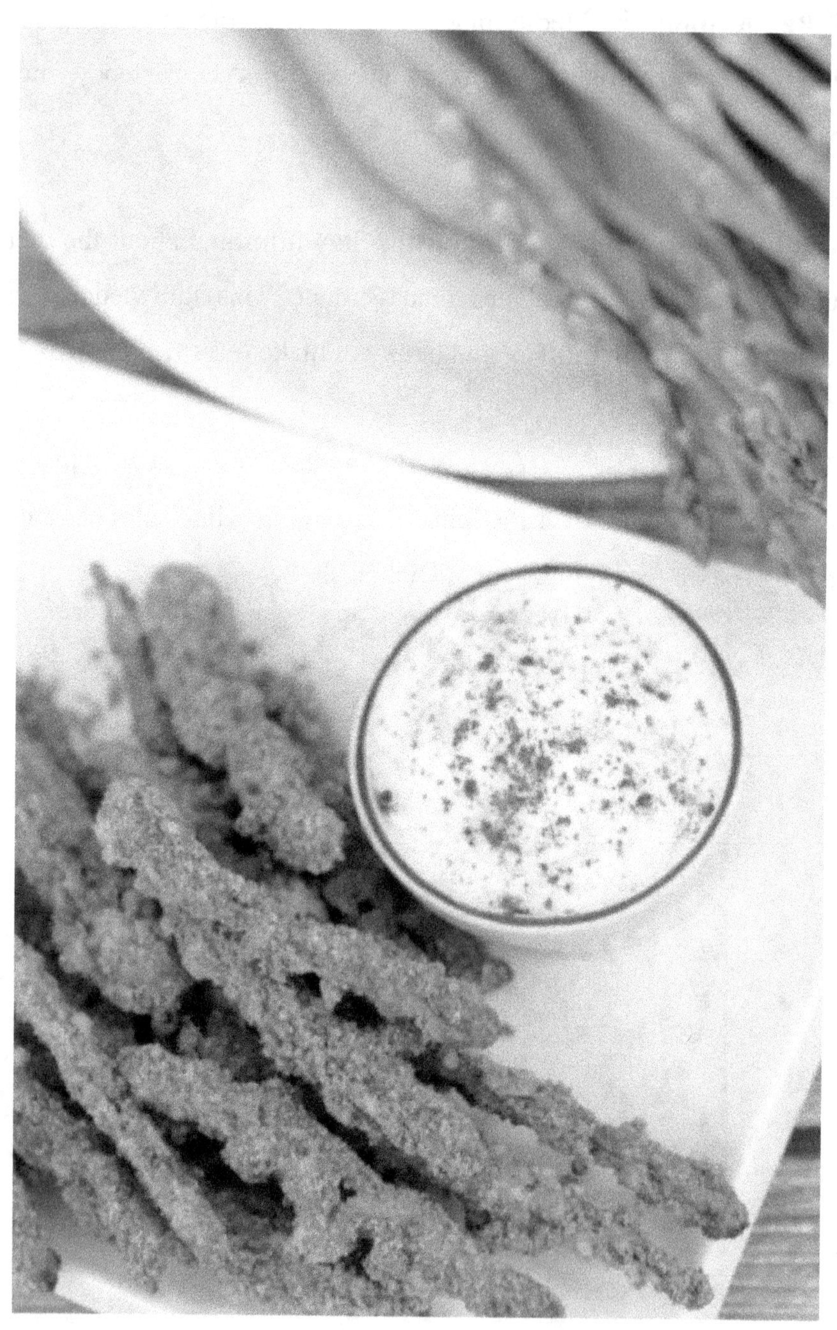

12. CONCLUSION

The Journey Ahead with the Mediterranean Diet

Embracing the Mediterranean Diet for Type 2 Diabetes is a journey towards improved health and well-being.

1. Lifelong Commitment: This diet is more than a temporary eating plan; it's a lifelong commitment to healthy living. The benefits extend beyond blood sugar control, offering improved heart health, weight management, and overall wellness.

2. Adaptability and Flexibility: The diet's adaptability makes it sustainable. You can adjust it based on personal preferences, cultural backgrounds, and seasonal availability of foods.

3. Continuous Learning and Experimentation: Stay curious and open to trying new foods and recipes. The Mediterranean diet is diverse, and exploring its range can keep the journey interesting and enjoyable.

4. Integrating Diet with Lifestyle: Remember, the diet is most effective when combined with other healthy lifestyle practices like regular physical activity, stress management, and social connections.

5. Celebrating Food and Life: The diet emphasizes the enjoyment of food and the importance of sharing meals with others, aligning eating habits with joy and social interaction.

As you continue with the Mediterranean Diet for Type 2 Diabetes, view it as a positive, enriching path that offers numerous benefits for your health and quality of life.

Final Tips and Encouragement

As you embark on this journey with the Mediterranean Diet for Type 2 Diabetes, here are some final tips and words of encouragement:

1. Persistence is Key: Change takes time, and persistence is essential. Embrace each step of this journey with positivity.

2. Celebrate Small Wins: Every healthy choice is a victory. Celebrate these moments to stay motivated.

3. Stay Informed: Continuously educate yourself about diabetes management and the Mediterranean diet. Knowledge is a powerful tool in this journey.

4. Seek Support: Don't hesitate to reach out to healthcare professionals, support groups, or online communities for guidance and support.

5. Remember the Benefits: Keep in mind the numerous health benefits this diet offers, from improved blood sugar levels to better heart health.

6. Enjoy the Process: Find joy in preparing and eating wholesome foods. Let the diet be a path to discovering new flavors and dishes.

7. Stay Flexible: Adapt the diet to fit your lifestyle and needs. Flexibility ensures long-term adherence.

8. Believe in Yourself: Have confidence in your ability to make positive changes for your health.

Remember, the Mediterranean Diet for Type 2 Diabetes is not just about food; it's a holistic approach to a healthier, happier life. You're making a wonderful choice for your well-being. Stay strong, stay inspired, and embrace the journey ahead.

www.ingramcontent.com/pod-product-compliance
Lightning Source LLC
Chambersburg PA
CBHW050825260726
48660CB00004B/1608